AF788734

CONTENTS

CONTENTS

QUICKENING THE PACE OF RESEARCH IN PROTECTING AGAINST ANTHRAX AND OTHER BIOLOGICAL TERRORIST AGENTS: A LOOK AT TOXIN INTERFERENCE

HEARING

BEFORE THE

COMMITTEE ON GOVERNMENT REFORM HOUSE OF REPRESENTATIVES

ONE HUNDRED SEVENTH CONGRESS

SECOND SESSION

FEBRUARY 28, 2002

Serial No. 107–64

Printed for the use of the Committee on Government Reform

Available via the World Wide Web: http://www.gpo.gov/congress/house
http://www.house.gov/reform

U.S. GOVERNMENT PRINTING OFFICE

79–590 PDF WASHINGTON : 2002

For sale by the Superintendent of Documents, U.S. Government Printing Office
Internet: bookstore.gpo.gov Phone: toll free (866) 512–1800; DC area (202) 512–1800
Fax: (202) 512–2250 Mail: Stop SSOP, Washington, DC 20402–0001

COMMITTEE ON GOVERNMENT REFORM

DAN BURTON, Indiana, *Chairman*

BENJAMIN A. GILMAN, New York
CONSTANCE A. MORELLA, Maryland
CHRISTOPHER SHAYS, Connecticut
ILEANA ROS-LEHTINEN, Florida
JOHN M. McHUGH, New York
STEPHEN HORN, California
JOHN L. MICA, Florida
THOMAS M. DAVIS, Virginia
MARK E. SOUDER, Indiana
STEVEN C. LATOURETTE, Ohio
BOB BARR, Georgia
DAN MILLER, Florida
DOUG OSE, California
RON LEWIS, Kentucky
JO ANN DAVIS, Virginia
TODD RUSSELL PLATTS, Pennsylvania
DAVE WELDON, Florida
CHRIS CANNON, Utah
ADAM H. PUTNAM, Florida
C.L. "BUTCH" OTTER, Idaho
EDWARD L. SCHROCK, Virginia
JOHN J. DUNCAN, Jr., Tennessee
——— ———

HENRY A. WAXMAN, California
TOM LANTOS, California
MAJOR R. OWENS, New York
EDOLPHUS TOWNS, New York
PAUL E. KANJORSKI, Pennsylvania
PATSY T. MINK, Hawaii
CAROLYN B. MALONEY, New York
ELEANOR HOLMES NORTON, Washington, DC
ELIJAH E. CUMMINGS, Maryland
DENNIS J. KUCINICH, Ohio
ROD R. BLAGOJEVICH, Illinois
DANNY K. DAVIS, Illinois
JOHN F. TIERNEY, Massachusetts
JIM TURNER, Texas
THOMAS H. ALLEN, Maine
JANICE D. SCHAKOWSKY, Illinois
WM. LACY CLAY, Missouri
DIANE E. WATSON, California
STEPHEN F. LYNCH, Massachusetts
———
BERNARD SANDERS, Vermont (Independent)

KEVIN BINGER, *Staff Director*
DANIEL R. MOLL, *Deputy Staff Director*
JAMES C. WILSON, *Chief Counsel*
ROBERT A. BRIGGS, *Chief Clerk*
PHIL SCHILIRO, *Minority Staff Director*

QUICKENING THE PACE OF RESEARCH IN PROTECTING AGAINST ANTHRAX AND OTHER BIOLOGICAL TERRORIST AGENTS: A LOOK AT TOXIN INTERFERENCE

THURSDAY, FEBRUARY 28, 2002

HOUSE OF REPRESENTATIVES,
COMMITTEE ON GOVERNMENT REFORM,
Washington, DC.

The committee met, pursuant to notice, at 10:10 a.m., in room 2154, Rayburn House Office Building, Hon. Dan Burton (chairman of the committee) presiding.

Present: Representatives Burton, Morella, Shays, Horn, Weldon, Waxman, Maloney, Norton, Cummings, Kucinich, Tierney, and Schakowsky.

Staff present: Kevin Binger, staff director; Mark Corallo, director of communications; S. Elizabeth Clay, professional staff member; Robert A. Briggs, chief clerk; Robin Butler, office manager; Elizabeth Crane and Michael Layman, legislative assistants; Elizabeth Frigola, deputy communications director; Joshua E. Gillespie, deputy chief clerk; Corinne Zaccagnini, systems administrator; Sarah Despres and David Rapallo, minority counsels; Ellen Rayner, minority chief clerk; and Jean Gosa, minority assistant clerk.

Mr. BURTON. A quorum being present, the Committee on Government Reform will come to order.

We have other Members who will be coming shortly. Mr. Waxman, the ranking minority member, is on his way, and Dr. Weldon I think is on his way as well.

I ask unanimous consent that all Members' and witnesses' opening statements be included in the record. Without objection, so ordered.

I ask unanimous consent that all articles, exhibits, and extraneous or tabular material referred to be included in the record. Without objection, so ordered.

In today's hearing we're continuing to look at how we can protect Americans against biological terrorism, primarily how to protect people from anthrax. Last fall, on the heels of the tragedy of September 11th and the loss of thousands of innocent lives, America was once again thrown into turmoil and fear. Our postal system was used to send anthrax spores through the mail. As a result, a small child contracted anthrax after attending a birthday party. Through this cowardly act, five innocent lives were lost.

We were caught totally unprepared. Government officials were forced to admit that there were serious holes in our treatment approach. They were forced to admit that our knowledge about how to treat anthrax is very limited. Right now we have two approaches. The first is the anthrax vaccine. The second is with antibiotics, and neither one is totally satisfactory.

We've spent a long time looking at the problems with the anthrax vaccine at the Defense Department. There's been a high rate of adverse events. The Department has never wanted to admit this. We have had military members in top physical condition come before the committee who became very ill shortly after receiving the vaccine. Pilots and other members of flight crews became so ill that they were grounded as a result of being forced to take the vaccine. Many of those who became ill were told it was not related to the vaccine, and they sometimes had to fight to receive adequate medical attention. Compounding that problem, it isn't clear at all that the vaccine will protect those that we have talked about against the known strains of anthrax.

I was a little disturbed earlier this year when postal employees and congressional staff were being offered the anthrax vaccine. Our health officials were really downplaying the problems with adverse events to those shots. I think they were either misinformed or they weren't being as candid as they should have been with the Congress. The postal workers and the congressional staff definitely weren't being given the facts about the problems at the Defense Department, and I don't think that's acceptable.

The antibiotics appear to be effective, but they are pretty strong, and they have to be taken for several months. Antibiotics can have some unpleasant side effects that make it difficult for some people to take this for an extended period.

So it's clear that we need to keep doing more research to better develop treatments that will deal with this problem. One of the most promising new treatments being developed is known as an "anti-toxin" treatment. That's what we're going to hear about today from our illustrious panel.

Anti-toxin treatments would stop anthrax spores from injecting toxins into human cells. According to many medical experts, this type of treatment holds tremendous promise. One of the things I want to do is to make sure we're directing enough research funding into this area.

Finding better treatments like anti-toxins is vital. Colonel Arthur Friedlander, a witness on today's second panel, is a senior scientist at the U.S. Army Medical Research Institute of Infectious Diseases at Fort Detrick. He has been part of the Army's anthrax biological defense program for a long time. In an article published in the journal Nature last year, Dr. Friedlander outlined a three-pronged approach to tackling the anthrax disease.

First, vaccination to prevent bacterial infection in the first place; second, antibiotics to attack infection if it occurs, and, third, anti-toxin treatments for the bacterium's toxic effects.

In order to develop effective anti-toxin treatments, it is important for scientists to understand how anthrax kills cells. Anthrax toxin, which is the dominant virulence factor of the anthrax bacteria, consists of three proteins. These three proteins—protective antigen, edema factor, and lethal factor—are all essential elements in what takes place when anthrax attacks cells.

I hope I pronounced that correctly—a senior investigator from the National Institute of Dental and Cranial Facial Research of the National Institutes of Health, is also testifying today. Dr. Leppla is part of a research team that identified how the lethal factor produced by anthrax spores kills cells.

Research, while competitive in nature, is often a team effort. This is especially important as we look at developing anti-toxin treatments. Research teams led by Dr. John Young of the University of Wisconsin and Dr. John Collier from Harvard Medical School began collaboration several years ago on the anthrax toxin research. They are both here today to explain their research and the role it may play in developing an anthrax anti-toxin.

I am pleased that Dr. Robert Smith could be with us today. He is the holder of 37 United States and foreign patents. Dr. Smith has made significant contributions to science. He is a professor emeritus of the University of California and a former section leader and senior biologist with the Lawrence Livermore National Laboratory.

Dr. Smith has given his career to improving our understanding of enzyme systems and monoclonal antibodies. In 1977, Dr. Smith founded Enzyme System Products in Livermore, CA to provide synthetic substrates and inhibitors to the scientific community. Dr. Smith will outline a proposal to protect against inhalation anthrax by inhibiting the furin enzyme on the surface of cells in the lung.

In addition to these attributes that Dr. Smith has, he's also the father of my son-in-law, who is with us today, and that makes him even more important. Don't you think that's interesting? Yes, I thought that was very interesting.

Dr. Gary Thomas, a senior scientist at Vollum Institute of Portland, OR, is a leading expert on human furin enzyme systems and has coauthored several papers with Dr. Leppla. He will explain how their research is contributing to our search for an anthrax anti-toxin.

As we move forward in looking at new treatments for biological terrorism agents, the role of advanced computer technology becomes increasingly important. Dr. Rodney Balhorn of the Lawrence Livermore National Laboratories will detail the role of our National Laboratories in developing treatments for anthrax.

We've brought together a prestigious group of experts. Today we will hear how this research is progressing. We will hear how we might achieve our goal of developing safe and effective treatments for our military population, first responders, and all Americans. The President's fiscal year 2003 budget calls for $5.9 billion to defend against biological terrorism, $2.4 billion of which is for scientific research.

This hearing will highlight one area in which, if we quicken the pace of the research, we may have products developed that can protect the public in a few years rather than the 12 to 15 years it is typically going to take. We don't have 12 to 15 years to wait. If we use just a small portion of the $2.4 billion this year on looking at toxin interference, we will be a lot closer to having a safe, effective, and scientifically validated treatment approach available.

I want to thank all of our witnesses for being here today. The hearing record will remain open until March 15 to allow for written submissions to the record.

[The prepared statement of Hon. Dan Burton follows:]

Opening Statement
of
Chairman Dan Burton
Committee on Government Reform

Hearing

"Quickening the Pace of Research in Protecting Against Anthrax and Other Biological Terrorist Agents - A Look at Toxin Interference."

February 28, 2001
10:00 am
2154 Rayburn House Office Building
Washington, DC

In today's hearing we are continuing to look at how we protect Americans against biological terrorism – primarily how to protect people from anthrax. Last fall, on the heels of the tragedy of September 11 and the loss of thousands of innocent lives, America was once again thrown into turmoil and fear. Our postal system was used to send anthrax spores through the mail. As a result, a small child contracted cutaneous anthrax after attending a birthday party. Through this cowardly act, five innocent lives were lost.

We were caught totally unprepared. Government officials were forced to admit that there were serious holes in our treatment approach. They were forced to admit that our knowledge about how to treat anthrax is very limited. Right now we have two approaches. The first is the anthrax vaccine. The second is with antibiotics. Neither one is totally satisfactory.

We've spent a long time looking at the problems with the anthrax vaccine at the Defense Department. There's been a high rate of adverse events. The Department has never wanted to admit this. We had military members in top physical condition that became ill shortly after receiving the vaccine. Pilots and other members of flight crews became so ill that they were grounded as a result of being forced to take the vaccine. Many of those who became ill were told it wasn't related to the shots. And they sometimes had to fight to receive adequate medical attention.

Compounding that problem -- it isn't clear at all that this vaccine will protect against all the known strains of anthrax.

I was a little disturbed earlier this year when postal employees and Congressional staff were being offered the anthrax vaccine. Our health officials were really downplaying the problems with adverse events to these shots. I think they were either misinformed, or they weren't being as candid as they should have been. The postal workers and Congressional staff definitely weren't being given all the facts about the problems at the Defense Department, and I don't think that's acceptable.

The antibiotics appear to be effective. But they are pretty strong, and have to be taken for several months. Antibiotics can have some unpleasant side effects that make it difficult for some people to take for this extended period.

So it's clear that we need to keep doing more research to develop better treatments. One of the most promising new treatments being developed is known as an "anti-toxin" treatment. That's what we're going to hear about today. Anti-toxin treatments would stop anthrax spores from injecting toxins into human cells. According to many medical experts, this type of treatment holds tremendous promise. One of the things I want to do is make sure we're directing enough research funding into this area.

Finding better treatments like anti-toxins is vital. Colonel Arthur Friedlander, a witness on today's second panel, is a senior scientist at the U.S. Army Medical Research Institute of Infectious Diseases at Ft. Detrick. He has been part of the Army's anthrax biological defense program for a long time. In an article published in the journal *Nature* last year, Dr. Friedlander outlined a three-pronged approach to tackling anthrax disease:

(1)Vaccination to prevent bacterial infection in the first place;
(2)Antibiotics to attack infection if it occurs, and
(3)Anti-toxin treatments for the bacterium's toxic effects.

In order to develop effective anti-toxin treatments, it is important for scientists to understand how anthrax kills cells. Anthrax toxin, which is the dominant virulence factor of the anthrax bacteria, consists of three proteins. These three proteins - protective antigen, edema factor, and lethal factor - are all essential elements in what takes place when anthrax attacks cells.

Dr. Stephen Leppla, a senior investigator from the National Institute of Dental and Cranial Facial Research of the National Institutes of Health is also testifying today. Dr. Leppla is part of a research team that identified how the lethal factor produced by anthrax spores kills cells.

Research, while competitive in nature, is often a team effort. This is especially important as we look at developing anti-toxin treatments. Research teams lead by Dr. John Young at the University of Wisconsin and Dr. John Collier from Harvard Medical School began collaboration several years ago on the anthrax toxin research. They both are here today to explain their research and the role it may play in developing an anthrax anti-toxin.

I am pleased that Dr. Robert Smith could be with us today. He is the holder of 37 U.S. and foreign patents. Dr. Smith has made significant contributions to science. He is a Professor Emeritus of the University of California and former section leader and senior biologist with the Lawrence Livermore National Laboratory. Dr. Smith has given his career to improving our understanding of enzyme systems and monoclonal antibodies. In 1977, Dr. Smith founded Enzyme System Products in Livermore, California to provide synthetic substrates and inhibitors to the scientific community. Dr. Smith will outline a proposal to protect against inhalation anthrax by inhibiting the Furin enzyme on the surface of cells in the lung.

Dr. Gary Thomas, a senior scientist at the Vollum Institute in Portland, Oregon, is a leading expert on human furin enzyme systems and has coauthored several papers with Dr. Leppla. He will explain how their research is contributing to our search for an anthrax anti-toxin.

As we move forward in looking at new treatments for biological terrorism agents, the role of advanced computer technology becomes increasingly important. Dr. Rodney Balhorn of the Lawrence Livermore National Laboratories will detail the role of our national laboratories in developing treatments for anthrax.

We've brought together a prestigious group of experts. Today we will hear how this research is progressing. We will hear how we might achieve our goal of developing safe and effective treatments for our military population, first responders, and all Americans. The President's fiscal year 2003 budget calls for $5.9 billion to defend against biological terrorism -- $2.4 billion of which is for scientific research.

This hearing will highlight one area in which, if we quicken the pace of the research, we may have products developed that can protect the public in a few years rather than the12 to15 years it typically takes. We don't have 12 to 15 years to wait. If we use just a small portion of the 2.4 billion dollars this year on looking at toxin interference, we will be a lot closer to having a safe, effective and scientifically validated treatment approach available.

I want to thank of our witnesses for being here today. The hearing record will remain open until March 15 to allow for written submissions to the record.

Mr. BURTON. Mr. Waxman, welcome.

Mr. WAXMAN. Thank you very much, Mr. Chairman. Thanks for holding this hearing.

In the aftermath of September 11th, there has been increasing attention paid to the country's preparedness to deal with the bioterror attack. In October of last year, the situation became even more urgent when a terrorist began mailing letters that contained finely milled and extremely dangerous anthrax, threatening the lives of postal workers and anyone else who could have come into contact with these potentially lethal spores.

This experience underscored the need for the country to increase its preparedness for a terror attack. One important response is to search for new potential treatments and methods of prevention. I am pleased that we will hear today from scientists who are looking at new ways to protect people from anthrax, and I look forward to hearing about how their research could impact on protection from and treatment of other diseases as well.

While having better protection from anthrax is an important component of bioterrorism preparedness, we must also recognize that anthrax is just one of many bioterrorism threats. We must commit ourselves to developing a comprehensive safety net that protects Americans from all threats to the maximum extent possible. This is an ambitious undertaking for our Nation's public health system.

Hearings like this are an important part of the process, but we will also need strong leadership from the administration. With Dr. Jeffrey Koplan's recent announcement that he will be stepping down as the Director of the Centers for Disease Control and Prevention, there are four critical public health jobs that are unfilled. These jobs include the Director of the CDC, Commissioner of the Food and Drug Administration, Director of the National Institutes of Health, and the Surgeon General. Together, these positions are the backbone of our national leadership for health emergencies. They need to be filled by leaders in public health. I hope that the President will see to that as soon as possible.

I thank the witnesses for coming today. I look forward to their testimony.

Thank you, Mr. Chairman.

[The prepared statement of Hon. Henry A. Waxman follows:]

ONE HUNDRED SEVENTH CONGRESS

Congress of the United States

House of Representatives

COMMITTEE ON GOVERNMENT REFORM

2157 RAYBURN HOUSE OFFICE BUILDING

WASHINGTON, DC 20515–6143

MAJORITY (202) 225–5074
FACSIMILE (202) 225–3974
MINORITY (202) 225–5051
TTY (202) 225–6852

www.house.gov/reform

Statement of Rep. Henry A. Waxman
Hearing on "Quickening the Pace of Research in Protecting Against Anthrax and Other Biological Terrorist Agents - A Look at Toxin Interference"
February 28, 2002

In the aftermath of September 11, there has been increasing attention paid to the country's preparedness to deal with a bioterror attack. In October of last year, the situation became even more urgent when a terrorist began mailing letters that contained finely milled and extremely dangerous anthrax, threatening the lives of postal workers and anyone else who could have come into contact with these potentially lethal spores.

This experience underscored the need for the country to increase its preparedness for a terror attack. One important response is to search for new potential treatments and methods of prevention. I am pleased that we will hear today from scientists who are looking at new ways to protect people from anthrax and I look forward to hearing about how their research could impact on protection and treatment from other diseases as well.

While having better protection from anthrax is an important component of bioterrorism preparedness, we must also recognize that anthrax is just one of many bioterrorism threats. We must commit ourselves to developing a comprehensive safety net that protects Americans from all threats to the maximum extent possible. This is an ambitious undertaking for our nation's public health system.

Hearings like this are an important part of the process, but we also need strong leadership from the Administration. With Dr. Jeffrey Koplan's recent announcement that he will be stepping down as director of the Centers for Disease Control and Prevention, there are four critical public health jobs that are unfilled. These jobs include the Director of the CDC, Commissioner of FDA, Director of NIH, and Surgeon General. Together, these positions are the backbone of national leadership for health emergencies. They need to be filled by leaders in public health.

I thank the witnesses for coming today and I look forward to their testimony.

Mr. BURTON. Thank you, Mr. Waxman. Mr. Shays.

Mr. SHAYS. Thank you, Mr. Chairman. Thank you for holding this hearing, and I welcome our panelists and our guests.

The global war against biological terrorism is also being waged at cellular and molecular levels. Research into the chemical and mechanical processes of anthrax infection, research tragically aided by the recent mail-borne attacks, points the way to a better vaccine, better antibiotic regimes, and new treatments to block the deadly toxins produced by the blooming bacteria.

A sharper focus on development of anti-toxins is warranted, some might say overdue, because anthrax has long been acknowledged as the most likely biological weapon threat. As this committee found in our oversight report 2 years ago, the current anthrax vaccine may cause serious adverse reactions in some, and it is not approved for use by children, the elderly, or pregnant women. Prolonged administration of broad-spectrum antibiotics can also cause untoward health effects, both in individuals and in terms of the public health threat of resistant organisms.

So effective treatments to shortcircuit the biochemical roots of anthrax toxicity are a missing element in our medical counterterrorism arsenal. Today's testimony will help us understand the status and potential of research into anthrax anti-toxins and the role new treatments might play in national preparedness against biological attacks.

So thank you again for having this hearing.

[The prepared statement of Hon. Christopher Shays follows:]

ONE HUNDRED SEVENTH CONGRESS

Congress of the United States

House of Representatives

COMMITTEE ON GOVERNMENT REFORM

2157 RAYBURN HOUSE OFFICE BUILDING

WASHINGTON, DC 20515–6143

MAJORITY (202) 225–5074
FACSIMILE (202) 225–3974
MINORITY (202) 225–5051
TTY (202) 225–6852

www.house.gov/reform

SUBCOMMITTEE ON NATIONAL SECURITY, VETERANS AFFAIRS,
AND INTERNATIONAL RELATIONS
Christopher Shays, Connecticut
Chairman
Room B-372 Rayburn Building
Washington, D.C. 20515
Tel: 202 225-2548
Fax: 202 225-2382
GROC.NS@mail.house.gov
http://www.house.gov/reform/ns/

Statement of Rep. Christopher Shays
February 28, 2002

The global war against biological terrorism is also being waged at cellular and molecular levels. Research into the chemical and mechanical processes of anthrax infection – research tragically aided by the recent mail-borne attacks – points the way to a better vaccine, better antibiotic regimes and new treatments to block the deadly toxins produced by the blooming bacteria.

A sharper focus on development of antitoxins is warranted, some might say overdue, because anthrax has long been acknowledged as the most likely biological weapons threat. As this committee found in our oversight report two years ago, the current anthrax vaccine may cause serious adverse reactions in some, and it is not approved for use by children, the elderly or pregnant women. Prolonged administration of broad-spectrum antibiotics can also cause untoward health effects, both in individuals and in terms of the public health threat of resistant organisms. So effective treatments to short-circuit the biochemical routes of anthrax toxicity are a missing element in our medical counterterrorism arsenal.

Today's testimony will help us understand the status and potential of research into anthrax antitoxins, and the role new treatments might play in national preparedness against biological attacks.

Mrs. MALONEY. Good morning, Mr. Chairman, and thank you so much for holding this——

Mr. BURTON. Mrs. Maloney is recognized for an opening statement.

Mrs. MALONEY. Thank you very much, and thank you for having this very important hearing.

The tragic deaths of five persons from inhalation anthrax, including Kathy Nguyen, who worked in my district at the Manhattan Eye, Ear and Throat Hospital, highlighted for the Nation our vulnerability to biological terrorism. These anthrax attacks not only scared the American people, but placed a severe strain on the public health system. As public servants and policymakers, we must do all we can to prevent bioterrorism. Additionally, it is imperative that we learn from the past, so that our citizens and our government can effectively respond to these crises in the future.

The men and women of our national security community have been battling terrorism for many years. As we will learn today, the Nation's scientists are critical to this fight. Our leading researchers are developing new approaches to preventing and treating many infectious agents, including anthrax infections.

In New York State our great institutions of higher learning are on the case. For instance, at Columbia University researchers at the College of Physicians and Surgeons and Mailman School of Public Health are studying the genetic composition of various infectious agents and providing training and assistance to Federal and State and local governments. Columbia is the home of one of the CDC's funded Centers for Public Health Preparedness. The Columbia Center is working closely with the New York City Department of Health to strengthen the connection between our academic medical centers and people on the front lines of public health. In August of last year, the Center trained over 700 public health nurses on what to do in the event of a major disaster, training which, unfortunately, came in all very handy during our crisis on September 11th.

At the Weill Medical College of Cornell University researchers are examining the human genes that are responsible for resistance to tuberculosis, to determine how these genes may protect an individual if exposed to anthrax infection. One additional example, at New York University's Medical Center, scientists have begun studies to examine interactions among the cells of the organism that causes anthrax to seek ways to inhibit their ability to infect people.

In addition, New York University researchers are using types of recombinant DNA technology to develop improved vaccines.

Although the tasks are daunting, with our country's scientists working to find better preventions and treatments, America can sleep better at night.

I look forward to the testimony today of the distinguished guests. Thank you.

[The prepared statement of Hon. Carolyn B. Maloney follows:]

STATEMENT OF CONGRESSWOMAN CAROLYN B. MALONEY

Committee on Government Reform
Full Committee Hearing

"Quickening the Pace of Research in Protecting Against Anthrax and Other Biological Terrorist Agents -- A Look at Toxin Interference"

February 28, 2002

Mr. Chairman and Ranking Member, thank you holding this hearing today.

The tragic deaths of five persons from inhalation anthrax – including Kathy Nguyen, who worked in my district at the Manhattan Eye, Ear and Throat Hospital -- highlighted for the nation our vulnerability to biological terrorism. These anthrax attacks not only scared the American people, but placed a severe strain on the public health system. As public servants and policy makers, we must do all we can to prevent bio-terrorism. Additionally, it is imperative that we learn from the past so that our citizens and our government can effectively respond to crises of the future.

The men and women of our national security community have been battling terrorism for many years. As we will learn today, the nation's scientists are critical to this fight, as well. Our leading researchers are developing new approaches to preventing and treating many infectious agents, including anthrax infections.

In New York state, our great institutions of higher learning are on the case. For instance, at Columbia University, researchers at the College of Physicians and Surgeons are studying the genetic composition of various infectious agents, conducting surveillance and diagnostics, and providing training and assistance to federal, state, and local governments.

Columbia is the home of one of the CDC-funded Centers for Public Heath Preparedness. The Columbia Center is working closely with the New York City Department of Health to strengthen the connection between our academic medical centers and people on the frontlines of public health. In August of last year, the Center trained over 700 public health nurses on what to do in the event of a major disaster, training which unfortunately came in all too handy.

At the Weill Medical College of Cornell University, researchers are examining the human genes that are responsible for resistance to tuberculosis to determine how these genes may protect an individual if exposed to anthrax infection.

One additional example: at New York University's Medical Center, scientists have begun studies to examine interactions among the cells of the organism that causes anthrax (B. anthracis) to seek ways to inhibit their communications. In addition, NYU researchers are using types of recombinant DNA technology to develop improved vaccines.

Although the tasks are daunting, with our country's scientists working to find better preventions and treatments, America can sleep better at night.

I look forward to the testimony of today's distinguished witnesses.

Thank you, Mr. Chairman.

#

Mr. BURTON. Mr. Tierney, do you have an opening statement?
Mr. TIERNEY. I will place it in the record, Mr. Chairman.
[The prepared statement of Hon. John F. Tierney follows:]

Statement of Rep. John F. Tierney House Government Reform Committee
Hearing on "Quickening the Pace of Research in Protecting Against Anthrax and Other Biological Terrorist Agents – A Look at Toxin Interference"
February 28, 2002

Thank you Mr. Chairman for calling this timely hearing. I look forward to hearing what our witnesses have to tell us about advances in the prevention and treatment of anthrax poison. At the same time, I am also interested in learning from them what type of security precautions the labs they work in have taken to prevent the theft or accidental loss of these highly lethal agents.

Since the initial discovery of anthrax sent through the mail last fall, law enforcement has scrambled to figure out who is responsible for this act of terrorism that killed 5 people. And yet, after 5 months, we still don't have any answers. All we have are more questions.

For example, how is it that security in our government's labs was so lax that no one knew which labs were experimenting with anthrax?

We also didn't know until recently which labs were experimenting with the Ames anthrax strain, which was the type sent in the mail.

Another question we don't have answers to is: which scientists were known to have experimented with anthrax toxins? According to the Washington Post, since last fall the FBI has conducted thousands of interviews and keeps a running list of people who are under scrutiny as possible suspects. And yet no individual has remained on the list for more than a month.

The government has clearly failed in its responsibility to maintain the security of our labs. Former employees at Fort Detrick, where much of the federal government's research on biological agents is done, report that there was little or no effort to account for dangerous substances. Instead of keeping track of scientists, the work they were doing and the times they were doing it, workers were allowed to freely pursue their experiments.

As a result, it was disclosed last month that 27 biological specimens had been reported missing by the Army labs in the early 1990s. The lost microbes included anthrax specimens and ebola specimens.

Now, law enforcement is forced to start from scratch as they try to find the individual responsible for the deaths of 5 people. Instead of referring to well-documented logs of researchers and their work, the FBI is reduced to sending letters to 40,000 members of the American Society of Microbiology, asking for help.

We should be ashamed of the lax security in our labs and learn from this tragedy. We need to ensure that strict security standards are in place in all labs, public and private, that are authorized to work with lethal toxins. We need to ensure that all scientists working in those labs have proper security clearance. And we need to ensure that we figure out quickly who is responsible for the anthrax letters sent last fall. At this point, there is nothing to stop the individual who sent those letters from sending more anthrax by mail and causing another public health emergency.

I look forward to hearing from our witnesses and welcome their testimony.

Mr. BURTON. Let me say, before I swear in the witnesses, that this is a very, very important hearing because we have just the two approaches that we talked about in dealing with the anthrax scare. This committee oversees the Postal Service, which has been severely threatened and impaired with the anthrax attacks that took place after September 11th. So we're very anxious to hear about your theories and alternatives to the conventional approaches to dealing with the anthrax threat.

I hope that you will do me a big favor. Knowing that most of us up here are not scientists or doctors, if you could speak in laymen's terms as much as possible, we would really appreciate it. When we get to the question-and-answer period, I think your answers probably will be more easily understood by us, but when you make your opening statements, which we're going to go to immediately, I hope that you'll try to remember that we want to understand as much as possible, and also the record, which will be reviewed by all the members of the committee, we want to make sure they understand it as well. So that if there is something that we should be doing in advising the administration on how to spend our scientific research dollars, we can do that with a little more knowledge than we have today.

So, with that, would you please stand so you can be sworn in.

[Witnesses sworn.]

Mr. BURTON. Be seated.

We normally have 5-minute opening statements, but I understand, because of the technical aspects of your testimony, it's going to take a little bit longer. So we'll be a little more lenient with our opening statements and give you the time that you require.

We will start with you, Dr. Smith.

STATEMENTS OF ROBERT SMITH, FOUNDER AND RESEARCH DIRECTOR, ENZYME SYSTEMS PRODUCT, LIVERMORE, CA; GARY THOMAS, SENIOR SCIENTIST AT VOLLUM INSTITUTE, PORTLAND, OR; JOHN COLLIER, PROFESSOR OF MICROBIOLOGY AND MOLECULAR GENETICS AT HARVARD MEDICAL SCHOOL, BOSTON, MA; AND JOHN A.T. YOUNG, PROFESSOR IN CANCER RESEARCH, MCARDLE LABORATORY FOR CANCER RESEARCH, UNIVERSITY OF WISCONSIN, MADISON, WI

Mr. SMITH. In the 1960's scientists struggled with the understanding of how the pancreatic islet cell hormone insulin was actually assembled into a two chain molecule with two connecting bridges. In 1967, Dr. Donald F. Steiner at the University of Washington published his findings that insulin was actually manufactured within the islet beta cells as a single chain protein, folded into a reverse position. This permits the formation of two disulfide-linking bridges. Only then is the connecting peptide proteolytically removed to yield biologically active insulin. The cleavage points are always the same, recognizing only a specific set of amino acids, and processed by a special enzyme called furin or converting enzymes, with the capability of converting an inactive proform-hormone into an active entity.

In 1972, as an employee of Eli Lilly and Co., I designed the first synthetic substrates to isolate the converting enzyme, and then to use that enzyme to obtain active insulin. My method of design was based on the active site modeling concept of two prominent researchers, Dr. Schecter and Dr. Berger of Israel. From this concept, I was successful in isolating a converting enzyme from human parathyroid tissue and converting proparathyroid bovine hormone into a functional hormone. The two completely distinct physiological events could be activated by a single pro forma mechanism suggesting the definition of a basic physiological axiom or principle.

Throughout the 1980's the scientific community believed that most protein hormones and enzymes are naturally synthesized in a proactive form. In the 1990's it was established that many cellular processes, including gene expression, cell cycle, programmed cell death or apoptosis, and intracellular protein targeting of bacteria and viruses are regulated by limited proteolysis of precursor proteins.

All of these functions are carried out by the proteolytic enzyme family of furins and convertases that are strategically localized within cells or on the cell surface. Furins within T lymphocytes are extremely important enzymes in the study because they play a major role in the processing of the glycoprotein of the HIV virus and the infectious strains of the Ebola virus. The presence of an activated furin enzyme on the cell surface of macrophages is necessary for a cell entry and a processing of bacterial toxins; most notable is anthrax.

Bacillus anthracis secretes three proteins to form toxic complexes at the surface of mammalian cells. The protective antigen is the principal component that is proteolytically activated from 83kDa-activated form to a 63kDa-activated entity, and the edema factor and the lethal factor, to form the toxic complex.

With this scientific background laid, researchers now have the understanding and the capability to design compounds that will function as protease inhibitor candidates that target specific enzymes, such as furins. Major pharmaceutical companies currently market protease inhibitor drugs that clinically stop, if only for a limited period of time, the progression of HIV infection and significantly reduce viral replication, except HIV protease inhibitors are generally directed to an enzyme endogenous to the genome of the virus and not to an enzyme of the candidate infectant cell. Consequently, the virus enzyme protein will inevitably mutate; thus, limiting the clinical effectiveness of the inhibitor drug.

When a person is exposed to Bacillus anthrax, the approach of treatment I propose is to inhibit the furin enzyme on the cell surface of the macrophages and the monocytes within the lung. Anthrax uses this furin enzyme to activate its protective antigen, enabling it to initiate a toxic state. Activation of the protective antigen by bacteria of anthrax is integral to the mechanisms of anthrax toxicity.

To be able to prevent the reduction in size of the PA 83kDa form to the 63kDa form would essentially enable the bacteria from entering the host designated cell and, most importantly, as a consequence, toxication could not occur. Theoretically, this can be accomplished with a sensitive, non-toxic, and specific protease inhibitor. The synthesis of such an inhibitor would prevent the protective antigen furin enzyme from functioning; thus, shutting down the enzyme before the toxic events could take place.

79-590 D-2

Is there a precedent that this furin inhibition mechanism would work as a first order of treatment? Yes, selective serine protease inhibitors to furins have been synthesized and used in cell cultures demonstrating the inability of the PA to be activated with the inhibitor present. The only commercially available furin inhibitors are Chloromethylketone derivatives that are strong alkalating agents, thus unacceptable. Because of their toxicity, they are useful only in establishing proof of principle and cannot be used as potential drug candidates.

I propose a new family of small molecular weight protease compounds: irreversible inhibitors, modeled around the furin activation cleavage site of the protective antigen with significant changes at the N-terminal and C-terminal ends. As a bioavailable agent, second-generation furin protease inhibitors are expected to meet the necessary criteria of low toxicity and high potency. There are strong scientific and financial arguments in defense of a protease inhibitor therapy over other types of therapeutic intervention for anthrax and certain viruses.

Time and the economics to develop these inhibitors are significantly less. Inhibitors could be extremely effective when following exposure to large masses of the population with very few side effects, adding to their desirability. Protease inhibitors can be manufactured economically and can be synthesized where different sequences are appropriate to various strains of toxins.

The mechanism of how HIV infects CD4 lymphocytes is dependent upon the furin processing of the gp160 viral protein at the REKR cleavage site, as shown on figure 6, to a gp120 protein and a 40 amino acid cutoff peptide. Inhibition of the gp160 processing has been reported to block syncytial formation and results in noninfective HIV virus particles. If it doesn't split, it won't infect, to paraphrase Johnny Cochran.

The findings published in science and medical journals indicate that furin inhibition is a feasible approach to preventing anthrax infection and demands rigorous exploration. Nevertheless, for the exploration to be practical, it will require the synthesis of new small molecular weight inhibitors that do not generate any residual cellular toxicity.

Until October of last year, my interests had been focused on a group of enzymes referred to as caspases. These enzymes have a propinquity to furins in a group designation, and one enzyme of the caspase family has significant control in the progression of cellular inflammation which parallels anthrax infection, identified as caspase 1.

In 1996, I designed an irreversible inhibitor referred to as Z-VAD-FMK for the study of Apoptosis, and to date over 800 publications utilizing this compound have appeared in leading scientific journals, from the references that you can see on the side panels, in the use of the possibility for treating of stroke, Parkinson's disease, Huntington's disease, spinal cord injury, and amyotrophic lateral sclerosis.

This same approach can bring success as an effective deterrent against bioterrorism through the design and synthesis of irreversible protease inhibitors that qualify as potential drug candidates.

Dr. Anthony Fauci stated January 14th at the National Press Club luncheon, “Most people don’t really think about research as an important component of the counter-bioterrorism issue, because in fact researchers are not first responders to the act. Yet research is a very important part of a comprehensive public health approach. I think that bioterrorism is in reality within the spectrum of what we are calling emerging and reemerging diseases where bioterrorism microbes are deliberately controlled for emerging and reemerging disease states.”

In conclusion, quickening the pace of research to lower the risk of death by bioterrorist attempts can be accomplished timely and economically through the design and synthesis of new and dynamic protease inhibitors, the vanguard of non-toxic and very specific compounds that target anthrax and the Ebola organisms.

Thank you very much.

[The prepared statement of Mr. Smith follows:]

ANTHRAX
"The Bigger Picture In Its Treatment"

Fig. 1

In the late 1960's, scientists struggled to understand how the pancreatic islet cell hormone insulin was actually assembled into a two chain molecule with two connecting bridges. In 1967, Dr. Donald F. Steiner at the Univ. of WA published his findings that insulin was actually manufactured within the islet B cells as a single chain protein, folded into a reverse position. This permits the formation of two disulfide-linking bridges. Only then is the connecting

Fig. 2

peptide proteolytically removed to yield biologically active insulin. The cleavage points are always the same, recognizing only a specific set of amino acids, and processed by a special enzyme called **Furin** or Converting enzyme, with the capability to convert an inactive proform-hormone into an active entity.

In 1972, as an employee of Eli Lilly and Company, I designed the first synthetic substrates to isolate the Converting enzyme, and then to use that

Fig. 3

enzyme to obtain active insulin. My method of design was based on the active site modeling concept of two prominent researchers, Schecter and Berger. From this concept I was successful in isolating a Converting enzyme from human parathyroid tissue and converting proparathyroid bovine hormone into a functional hormone. That two completely distinct physiological events could be activated by a single pro-forma mechanism suggested the definition of a basic physiological axiom or principal.

Throughout the 1980's the scientific community believed that most protein hormones and enzymes are naturally synthesized in a proactive form. In the

1990's it was established that many cellular processes including gene expression, cell cycle, embryogenesis, programmed cell death or apoptosis, endocrine/neural functions and intracellular protein targeting of bacteria and viruses are regulated by limited proteolysis of precursor proteins. All of these functions are carried out by the proteolytic enzyme families of **Furins** and Convertases that are strategically localized within cells or on the cell surface. **Furins** within T lymphocytes are **extremely important enzymes** to study because they play a major role in the processing of the glycoprotein envelope of many viruses such as human immuno-deficiency virus (HIV) and the infectious strains of the Ebola virus. The presence of the activated Furin enzyme on the cell surface of macrophages is necessary for a cell entry and the processing of bacterial toxins—most notable is **Anthrax.**

Fig. 4 Bacillus anthracis secretes three proteins to form toxic complexes at the surface of mammalian cells. The protective antigen is the central component that is proteolytically activated from 83kDa activated down to a 63kDa fragment that binds to the edema factor (EF) and a lethal factor (LF) to form the toxic complexes.

With this scientific groundwork laid researchers now have the understanding and capability to design compounds that will function as protease inhibitor-drug candidates that target specific enzymes (such as **furin**). Major pharmaceutical companies currently market protease inhibitor drugs that clinically **stop** (at least temporarily) the progression of HIV infection and significantly reduce viral replication. Except, HIV protease inhibitors are generally directed to an enzyme endogenous to the genome of the virus and not to an enzyme of the candidate infectant cell. Consequently, the virus enzyme protein will invariably mutate; thus limiting the clinical effectiveness of the inhibitor drug.

When a person is exposed to Bacillus anthracis, the approach of treatment that I propose is to inhibit the Furin enzyme on the cell surface of macrophages and monocytes within the lungs. Anthrax uses this Furin enzyme to activate its protective antigen, enabling it to initiate an infectious state. Activation of the protective antigen (PA63) of Bacillus anthracis is integral to the mechanism of anthrax toxicity.

To be able to prevent the reduction in size of the PA 83kDa form to the 63kDa form would essentially enable the bacteria protein from entering the host designated cells and **most importantly** as a consequence—**infection could not occur**. Theoretically, this can be accomplished with a sensitive, non-toxic and specific protease inhibitor. The synthesis of such an inhibitor would prevent the (protective antigen) Furin enzyme from functioning, (shutting the enzyme down before the toxin can infect).

Fig. 5

Is there a precedent that this Furin inhibition mechanism would work as a first order of treatment? Yes! Selective serine protease inhibitors to Furins have been synthesized and used in cell cultures demonstrating the inability of the PA to be activated with the inhibitor present. The only commercially available Furin inhibitors are Chloromethylketone derivatives that are strong alkalating agents, thus unacceptable. Because of their toxicity they are useful only in establishing **proof of principle** and cannot be used as potential drug candidates.

Fig. 7

I propose a new family of small molecular weight protease compounds. Irreversible inhibitors, modeled around the Furin activation cleavage site of the protective antigen with significant changes at the N-terminal and C-terminal ends. As a bioavailable agent, second generation Furin protease inhibitors are expected to meet the necessary criteria of low toxicity and high potency. There is strong scientific and financial arguments in defense of protease inhibitor therapy over other types of therapeutic intervention for Anthax and certain viruses. Time and the economics to develop these inhibitors are significantly less. Inhibitors could be extremely effective when following exposure to large masses of the population with very few side affects, adding to their desirability. Protease inhibitors can be manufactured economically and can be synthesized where different sequences are applicable to various strains of toxins.

Fig. 6

The mechanism of how HIV infects CD4 lymphocytes is dependent upon a Furin processing of the gp160 viral protein at the REKR cleavage site to gp120 and a 40 amino acid cut off peptide. Inhibition of gp160 processing has been reported to block syncytial formation and results in non-infective HIV viral particles. "If it doesn't split it won't infect" (Jonny Cochran) to paraphrase.

The findings published in science and medical journals indicate that Furin inhibition is a feasible approach to preventing anthrax infection and **demands** rigorous exploration. Nevertheless, for exploration to be practical it will require the synthesis of new small molecular weight inhibitors that do not generate any residual cellular toxicity.

Fig. 8 — Until October of last year my interests had been focused on a group of enzymes referred to as caspases. These enzymes have a propinquity to Furins in a group designation, and one enzyme of the caspase family has significant control in the progression of cellular inflammation which parallels anthrax infection; identified as caspase 1. In 1996, I designed an **irreversible** protease inhibitor referred to as Z-VAD-FMK for the study of

Fig. 9 — Apoptosis and to date over 800 publications utilizing this compound have appeared in leading scientific journals. **This same approach can bring success as an effective deterrent against bio-terriorism through the**

Fig. 10 — **design and synthesis of irreversible protease inhibitors that qualify as potential drug candidates.**

Dr. Anthony Fauci (Director of the National Institutes of Allergy and Infectious Diseases, of NIH), stated January 14th. at the National Press Club luncheon "Most people don't really think about research as an important component of the counter-bio-terrorism issue, because in fact researchers are not first responders to the act. Yet research is a very important part of a comprehensive public health approach. I think that bio-terrorism is in reality within the spectrum of what we call emerging and reemerging diseases where bio-terrorism microbes are deliberately controlled for emerging and reemerging disease states."

Fig. 11 — In conclusion, quickening the pace of research to lower the risk of death by bio-terriorist attempts can be accomplished **timely** and **economically** through the design and synthesis of new and dynamic protease inhibitors, the **vanguard** of non-toxic and very specific compounds that target anthrax and ebola micro-organisms.

Congress of the United States

House of Representatives

COMMITTEE ON GOVERNMENT REFORM

"Quickening the Pace of Research in Protecting Against Anthrax and Other Biological Terrorist Agents"

by

Dr. Robert E. Smith

February 28, 2002

Fig. 1 **Primary Structure of Human Proinsulin**

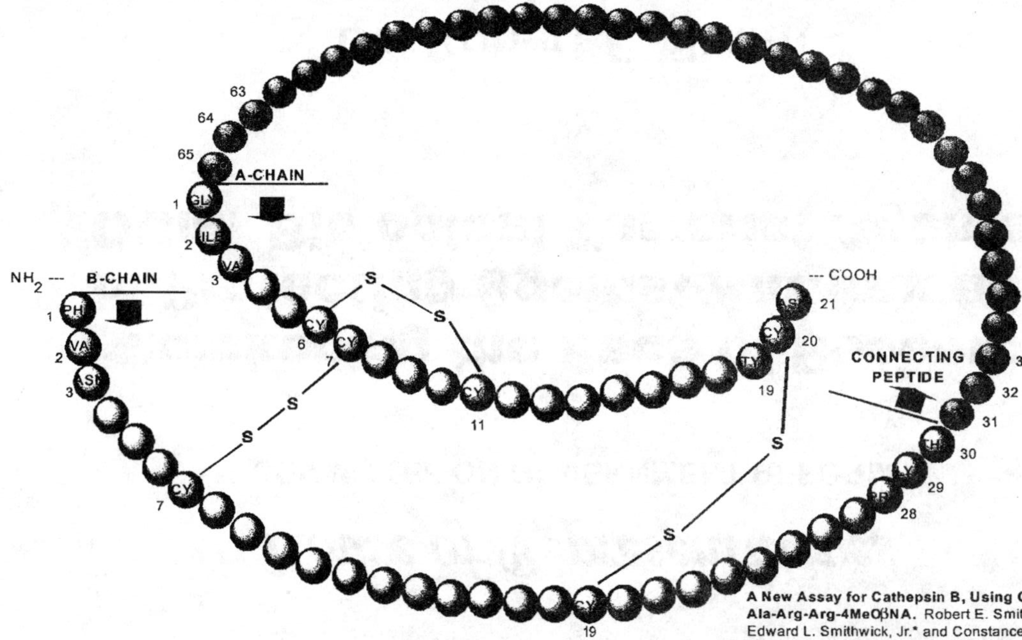

A New Assay for Cathepsin B, Using CBZ-Ala-Arg-Arg-4MeOβNA. Robert E. Smith, Edward L. Smithwick, Jr.* and Constance H. Allen. *Eli Lilly and Company. The Lilly Research Laboratories, Inidanapolis, Ind.*

Twenty-third Annual Meeting
Boston, Massachusetts
October 14 and 15, 1972

Fig. 2

Primary Structure of Human Insulin

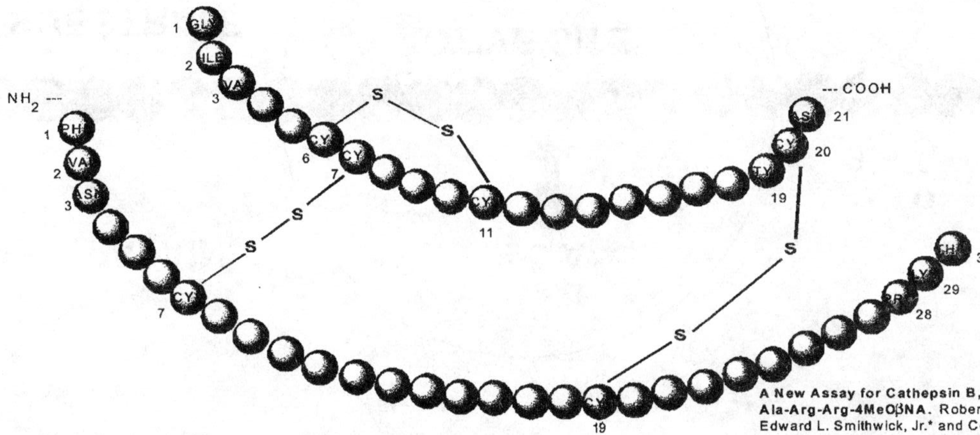

A New Assay for Cathepsin B, Using CBZ-Ala-Arg-Arg-4MeOβNA. Robert E. Smith, Edward L. Smithwick, Jr.* and Constance H. Allen. *Eli Lilly and Company. The Lilly Research Laboratories, Inidanapolis, Ind.*

Twenty-third Annual Meeting
Boston, Massachusetts
October 14 and 15, 1972

Fig. 3

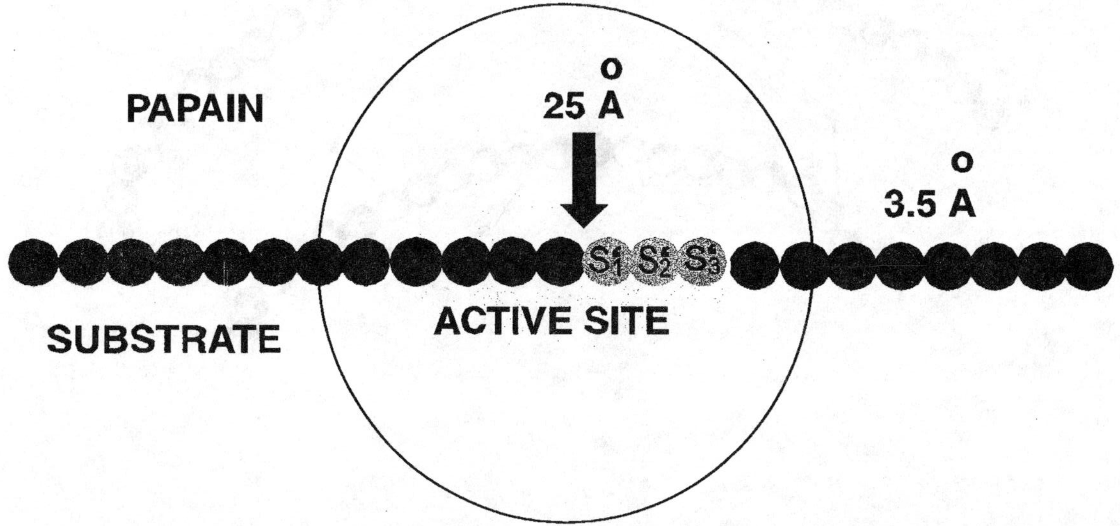

Fig. 4

Furin catalyzes activation of the anthrax toxin

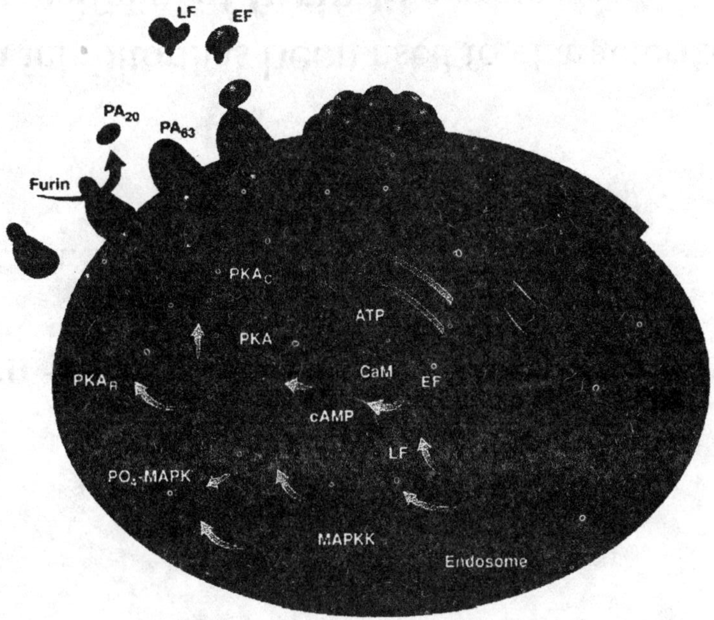

Fig. 5

Decanoyl – Arg – Val – Lys – Arg - chloromethylketone

Mol. Wt. 744.42 $C_{34}H_{66}ClN_{11}O_5$

This **furin** inhibitor has been used to characterize the specificity of **furin-like** proteases

Fig. 6

Table 1 Furin proteolytic activation sites.

			P_4	P_3	P_2	P_1			
Baterial toxins									
Anthrax toxin PA	N	S	**R**	K	**K**	**R**	|	S	T
Clostribium septicum α-toxin	K	R	**R**	G	**K**	**R**	|	S	V
Diphteria toxin	G	N	**R**	V	**R**	**R**	|	S	V
Proaerolysin	K	V	**R**	R	A	**R**	|	S	V
Pseudomonas exotoxin A	R	H	**R**	Q	P	**R**	|	G	W
Shiga toxin	A	S	**R**	V	A	**R**	|	M	A
Viral coat proteins									
Avian influenza HA (HSN1)	R	R	**R**	K	**K**	**R**	|	G	L
Borna disease virus	L	K	**R**	R	**R**	**R**	|	D	T
Cytomegalovirus gB	T	H	**R**	T	**R**	**R**	|	S	T
Ebola Zaire GP	G	R	**R**	T	**R**	**R**	|	E	A
Marburg	V	Y	**R**	R	**K**	**R**	|	S	I
Epstein-Barr virus gB	L	R	**R**	R	**R**	**R**	|	D	A
HIV-1 gp160	V	Q	**R**	E	**K**	**R**	|	A	V
Infectious bronchitis virus E2	T	R	**R**	F	**R**	**R**	|	S	I
Japan B encephalitis M	S	K	**R**	S	**R**	**R**	|	S	V
Measles virus F_o	S	R	**R**	H	**K**	**R**	|	F	A
Mumps	S	R	**R**	H	**K**	**R**	|	F	A
Respiratory-syncitial virus F	K	K	**R**	K	**R**	**R**	|	F	L
Rous sarcoma virus env	G	I	**R**	R	**K**	**R**	|	S	V
Yellow fever virus M	S	G	**R**	S	**R**	**R**	|	S	V

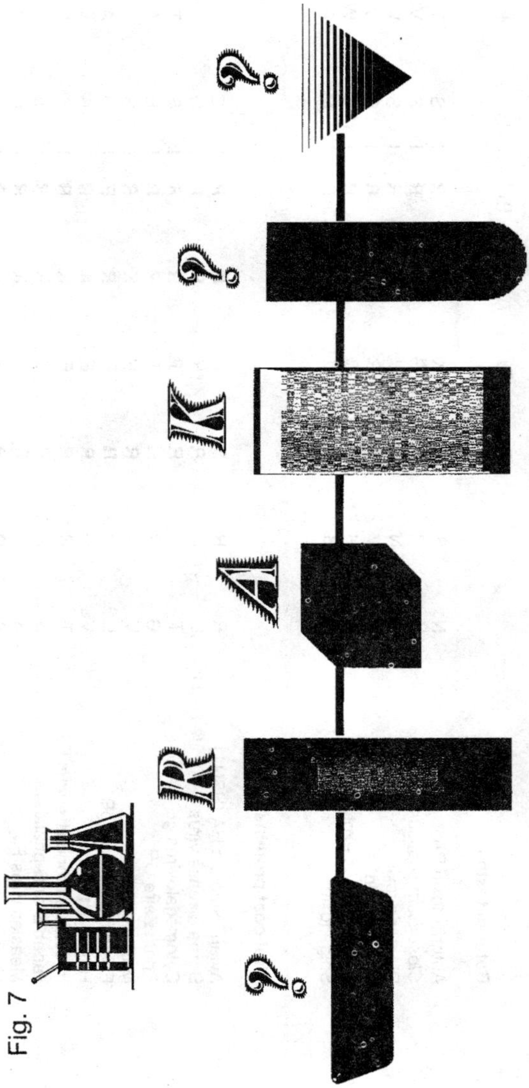

Fig. 7

Fig. 8

Caspase Inhibition Prevents Cardiac Dysfunction and Heart Apoptosis in a Rat Model of Sepsis

Remi Neviere, Harold Fauvel, Claude Chopin, Pierre Formstecher, and Philippe Marchetti

INSERM U459, Faculte de Medecine, EA 2689, Pavaillon Vancostenobel, Faculte de Medecine, and Departement de Physiologie, Faculte de Medecine, Lille Cedex, France

---

NEUROLOGICAL PROGRESS

Caspases as Treatment Targets in Stroke and Neurodegenerative Diseases

Jorg B. Schultz, MD, Michael Weller, MD, and Michael A. Moskowitz, MD

Ann Neurol 1999; 45:421-429

Neuroscience, Vol. 99, No. 2, pp. 333-342, 2000

FUNCTIONAL ROLE AND THERAPEUTIC IMPLICATIONS OF NEURONAL **CASPASE**-1 AND –3 IN A MOUSE MODEL OF TRAUMATIC SPINAL CORD INJURY

M. Li, V.O. Ona, M. Chen, M. Kaul, L. Tenneti, X. Zhang, P.E. Stieg, S.A. Lipton, and R.M. Friedlander

Neuroapoptosis Laboratory and Neurosurgical Service, Department of Surgery, Cerebrovascular and Neuroscience Research Institute, and Cardiovascular Division, Department of Medicine, Brigham and Women's Hospital, Harvard Medical School, Boston, MA 02115, USA

The Journal of Biological Chemistry
1999 by The American Society for Biochemistry and Molecular Biology, Inc.

Vol. 274, No. 33, Issue of August 13, pp. 23426-23436, 1999©
Printed in U.S.A.

Caspase-6 Role in Apoptosis of Human Neurons, Amyloidogenesis, and Alzheimer's Disease

(Received for publication, February 12, 1999, and in revised from, April 19, 1999)

Andrea LeBlanc, Hui Liu, Cynthia Goodyer, Catherine Bergeron, and Jennifer Hammond

Fig. 9

Caspase-3: A vulnerability factor and final effector in apoptotic death of dopaminergic neurons in Parkinson's disease

Andrease Hartmann, Stephane Hunot, Patrick P. Michel, Marie-Paule Muriel, Sheela Vyas, Baptiste A. Faucheux, Annick Mouatt-Prigent, Helene Turmel, Anu Srinivasan, Merle Ruberg, Gerard I. Evan, Yves Agid, and Etienne C. Hirsch

---

J. Neurosci 1999 Feb 1; 19(3):964-973

Mutant Huntingtin Expression in Clonal Striatal Cells: Dissociation of Inclusion Formation and Neuronal Survival by Caspase Inhibition.

Kim M, Lee HS, LaForet G, McIntyre C., Martin EJ, Chang P, Kim TW, Williams M, Reddy PH, Tagle D, Boyce FM, Won L, Heller A, Aronin N, DiFiglia M

Journal of Neuropathology and Experimental Neurology Vol 58, No.5

May 1999
pp. 459-471

Neuronal Death in Amyotrophic Lateral Sclerosis Is Apoptosis: Possible Contribution of a Programmed Cell Death Mechanism

Lee J. Marthin, PhD

Fig. 10

The Journal of Biological Chemistry
Vol. 267, No. 28, Issue of August 15, pp. 16396-16402 1992
Printed in U.S.A.

Human Furin Is a Calcium-dependent Serine Endoprotease That Recognizes the Sequence Arg-X-X-Arg and Efficiently Cleaves Anthrax Toxin Protective Antigen

(Received for publication, April 9, 1992)

Sean S. Molloy, Patricia A. Bresnahan, Stephen H. Leppla, Kurt R. Klimpel, and Gary Thomas

---

Proc. Natl. Acad. Sci. USA
Vol. 89, pp. 10277-10281, November 1992
Biochemistry

Anthrax toxin protective antigen is activated by a cell surface protease with the sequence specificity and catalytic properties of furin

(Bacillus anthracis/protein processing/paired basic residues/mutagenesis/consensus sequence)

Kurt R. Klimpel, Sean S. Molloy, Gary Thomas, and Stephen H. Leppla

---

Proc. Natl. Acad. Sci. USA
Vol. 95, pp. 5762-5767, May 1998
Microbiology

Processing of the Ebola virus glycoprotein by the proprotein convertase furin

(proteolytic processing)

Viktor E. Volchkov, Heinz Feldmann, Valentina A. Volchkova, and Hans-Dieter Klenk
Institut fur Virologie, Philipps-Universitat Marburg, 35011 Marburg, Germany

---

The Journal of Biological Chemistry
Vol. 276, No. 25, Issue of June 22, pp. 22090-22094, 2001

Printed in U.S.A.

A Dominant Negative Mutant of *Bacillus anthracis* Protective Antigen Inhibits Anthrax Toxin Action *in Vivo*

Received for publication, November 9, 2000, and in revised form, March 6, 2001
Published, JBC Papers in Press, March 16, 2001, DOI 10.1074/jbc.M010222200

Yogendra Singh, Hemant Khanna, Arun P. Chopra, and Varsha Mehra
From the Centre for Biochemical Technology, Mall Road, Delhi-110007, India

Fig. 11

If this mechanism of enzyme/inhibitor technology can be achieved it would make biological micro-organism warfare much less lethal and bio-terrorism less grievous.

Mr. BURTON. Thank you, Dr. Smith. When we get to the questions, I'll ask you some questions in laymen's terms that perhaps you can—because you were over my head a little bit there from time to time; in fact, most of the time. But I think I got the gist of what you were saying.

Our next panelist is Dr. Gary Thomas. He's a senior scientist at Vollum Institute in Portland, OR. Is that correct?

Mr. THOMAS. That's correct.

Mr. BURTON. You're recognized.

Mr. THOMAS. Well, Mr. Burton and other members of the committee, it's certainly an honor to be here today to summarize for you and explain——

Mr. BURTON. Can you pull your mic a little closer, sir? Thank you very much.

Mr. THOMAS [continuing]. To explain for you the role of furin in pathogen virulence and human disease. I have an overhead presentation that I'm not quite sure will work, but we'll give this a try, because it's slightly out of context from my written testimony, but we'll give it a try. If it doesn't work, we'll go back to my written testimony.

But, to begin with, the reprehensible bioterrorism plot following the September 11th World Trade Center tragedy intended to inflict countless deaths by disseminating the Bacillus anthracis spores throughout the U.S. mail. Eleven victims contracted the deadly lethal form of inhalation anthrax, leaving five of these victims to die within days following infection.

If I can have the next overhead, and one more. Now anthrax is a frightening pathogen, and the recent anthrax scare is eerily reminiscent of the near influenza pandemic that erupted in Hong Kong just 5 years ago, where a renegade pathogenic avian influenza virus jumped directly from birds to humans. Similar to the death rate that we experienced with the anthrax toxicity, 6 of the 18 persons clinically diagnosed with this bird flu were dead within 1 week.

Besides illustrating our vulnerability to the deadly microbes, is there a link between the anthrax and the "bird flu" outbreaks? Yes, clearly one link is the enzyme furin. So what is furin and how does it work?

Well, furin is an enzyme, and it's the type of enzyme called the protease, which does a very simple job. It cuts a larger protein and turns it into a smaller protein, but furin doesn't just cut any protein. It cuts a select group of proteins that contain within them a furin site.

If I can show the next overhead, please. Now this cleavage that occurs allows furin to generate from an inactive precursor protein, a smaller and biologically active molecule, and it's this active protein product, that is, the smaller, biologically active molecule, that is responsible for the damage that's inflicted by many pathogens.

Now, interestingly, the identification of the furin site was identified in collaboration with Dr. Steve Leppla, who is here as well, when we characterized the ability of furin to cleave the protective antigen component of the anthrax toxin 10 years ago.

Next slide, please. Now furin is a cellular enzyme, but it's probably over the last 10 to 12 years of research by my lab and other labs it's become recognized, I think, as really the Dr. Jekyll and Mr. Hyde of the South. There's certainly an important role that furin plays in embryogenesis, but in the adult there's a decidedly dark side of furin as well, and this is what I would like to share with you today.

Furin is certainly involved and is necessary for the activation not only of anthrax, but of many bacterial toxins, including pseudomonas toxins, shiga toxin, gangrene-forming toxins as well. Specifically with anthrax, we've heard about this already, and I'll summarize it quickly on the next slide, furin at the cell surface is responsible for the activation of the protective antigen component of anthrax, and that's a cleavage that turns protective antigen from an inactive molecule to an active molecule.

By activating the protective antigen component, protective antigen is able to deliver into the cell one of the two toxic factors, either the edema or lethal factor that you've explained, and you'll hear more about by the other panelists. That's what goes on to kill the cell. So, in fact, furin is the key to this pathway. We look at it as beginning this entire cascade that leads to cell death.

Next slide, please. Now furin is not only involved in the activation of many bacterial toxins, but it turns out a number of pathogenic viruses require this pathway as well. These include, for example, HIV, cytomegalovirus virus, respiratory syncytial virus, Ebola virus, yellow fever virus. There's a number of viruses that have envelope glycoproteins on their cell surface that must be cleaved to produce infectious progeny.

Not only is furin involved in pathogen activation, but furin plays a role in very detrimental diseases in humans as well. On the next two panels, it plays a role in rheumatoid arthritis and metastatic cancer. Now rheumatoid arthritis is activated—if I can also show the next slide, please—by furin's activation of a protease cascade that leads to the breakdown of cartilage in joints.

Now metastatic tumors—if you could go back one slide; I don't know if we can do that or not—in the bottom righthand panel of that slide is actually a biopsy section from a tumor. Furin turns out to play a prominent role in tumor metastasis, where furin is upregulated in many metastatic tumors. Shown in that panel in the bottom righthand corner of the slide, of the projection, is a biopsy from a patient, and that biopsy was stained for furin. You can see that the staining of that tumor is, in fact, increased for furin, and in fact furin levels correlate with the invasiveness of many metastatic tumors.

Well, because of furin's role in both pathogen activation and human disease, is it a target, a strategic target, for both bioterrorism and human disease. We think it is, and we think it is for several reasons. I think one of the prominent reasons is because Mother Nature tells us it's an excellent target.

Please, on the next slide. That is that we find that many pathogens that learn to exploit the furin pathway simply become more deadly. I think one of the classic examples that's been used is the Ebola virus itself. There are various islets of Ebola virus. One of them is called Reston. Now Reston is basically non-pathogenic in humans, and it's non-pathogenic in part because it doesn't know how to use the furin pathway, but there's other islets of Ebola virus that are much more deadly, like Ebola Zaire, on the next panel, please.

Ebola Zaire has mutated its glycoprotein to now use the furin pathway. Because it can use the furin pathway, it causes 90 percent fulminant disease and death in humans very rapidly.

Now is Ebola virus the only virus that has learned to use the furin pathway that causes such havoc on humans? No. In fact, on the next panel—in fact, why don't you stop there for just a second? That Hong Kong bird flu that jumped from birds directly to humans, one of the reasons it was capable of infecting and killing humans is because it learned how to use the furin pathway, this protease that we talked about earlier.

So can we develop furin inhibitors and can we block furin to use to our benefit? I think that we can. We have done this in an approach where we have generated a protein-based inhibitor, and this is shown on this slide here. It's an inhibitor that we call Alpha–1-PDX. Basically, Alpha–1-PDX, we pirated a scapold of a protein that's in all of our circulation called Alpha–1 antitrypsin, but we've simply put into this protein the furin site, so that furin will try to now recognize this inhibitor. This inhibitor, for lack of a better term, functions as a molecular mousetrap.

If you could show the next panel, please. In the next panel, furin will try to cleave this inhibitor—keep going; right there and stop—but instead of releasing from the enzyme, this inhibitor basically folds over the enzyme and traps it and it activates the enzyme. So, in fact, using this inhibitor, we've shown that we can simply control the levels of furin in cells, and that works to our advantage quite greatly for the ability to protect against a number of pathogens.

There's some key advantages to using this technology. Please, on the next slide. One is, in fact, that it is very potent. Second is that it is highly selective, and the third is in the acute toxicity studies that we have done so far, we see no toxicity.

So, actually, can this inhibitor block the furin pathway and protect against pathogens? Is this a novel approach to a broad-based therapeutic? We think it is.

On the next slide, some examples that will show you are, for example, HIV. As you know, HIV infects cells, and it needs to do this by using a protrusion on the envelope of the virus, which attaches to the cell and allows the virus to fuse with the cell. Now the protein that needs to be processed by furin, so that it becomes active and fusogenic requires the furin pathway. This is an envelope protein called gp160. Our inhibitor will block this processing, and by blocking this processing, block the production of infectious virus.

If you can show the next panel, what I'll show you are some cell culture studies that we've done just simply showing how this inhibitor will block the virus.

Well, for sake of time, we can skip ahead. I think just stay right there. I think we're fine.

Basically, we can block HIV because HIV uses the furin pathway. Now is this going to only work on HIV? No. It turns out that this inhibitor will block a number of viruses that require the furin pathway, including cytomegalovirus and measles virus, and we think by extension any number of other pathogen human viruses that simply require the furin pathway for their virulence.

Is it restricted to viruses? No. In fact, we can use this same type of technology to actually protect cells against bacterial toxins. An example that we use is pseudomonas toxin. We think because the anthrax toxin also requires the furin pathway in studies that we collaborated on with Dr. Leppla, we think that this type of technology leads us to a path that we could also protect against anthrax and other deadly toxins as well that require this pathway.

Now what about human disease? In fact, as I told you earlier a few minutes ago, in fact, furin is involved in tumor metastasis and plays a very ugly role in this process. How does it do this? Furin activates an enzyme cascade that leads to tumor metastasis.

If you could just keep going through these slides, this activation—part of this is not going to come up—but, basically, this activation leads to the ability of tumor cells to leave a localized place and spread throughout the body because they're able to secrete some proteases that allow them to degrade cell barriers.

What we find is that entire cascade starts with furin. What we found, in collaboration with Dr. Andres Klein-Szanto at the Fox Chase Cancer Center in Philadelphia, was that if we blocked that pathway, we can block cancer metastasis in a simple animal model. That's shown in the bottom lefthand corner of the slide here. It might be a little difficult to see, but, basically, he took an aggressive tumor cell and placed it in an animal. When he does this, that tumor cell will grow and will metastasize through the animal. If he treats that tumor cell with PDX, this inhibitor that we have, this first-generation inhibitor, in fact, it blocks tumor metastasis, and it's still encapsulated, which is shown in the middle bottom part of this panel.

Next slide, please. So is furin a novel target both against bioterrorism and disease? We think that it is. We think that its role in bacterial toxin activation, in the activation of millions of many pathogenic viruses, and also in human disease, I think strongly suggests that furin is an excellent target for the generation of broad-based therapeutics.

I think that together with the expertise of others at this hearing, we may, indeed, develop an exciting new strategy to protect against biological terrorist pathogens as well as debilitating human diseases. Thank you, sir.

[The prepared statement of Mr. Thomas follows:]

Congress of the United States
House of Representatives
Committee on Government Reform
The Honorable Dan Burton, Chairman

February 28, 2002

Testimony for the hearing "Quickening the Pace of Research in Protecting Against Anthrax an Other Biological Terrorist Agents – A Look at Toxin Interference."

"The role of furin in pathogen virulence and human disease"

by

Gary Thomas, Ph.D. Senior Scientist, Vollum Institute, OHSU, Portland, OR

The reprehensible bioterrorism plot following the September 11 World Trade Center tragedy intended to inflict countless deaths by disseminating *Bacillus anthracis* spores through the U.S. mail. As of December 2001, 22 persons were diagnosed with anthrax from contacting contaminated mail. Eleven of these cases were confirmed as the deadly inhalation anthrax, leaving five of these victims to die within days of their exposure [1, 2]. That the New Jersey and District of Columbia mail sorting facilities processed nearly 85 million pieces of mail on the days after the contaminated letters were sent to NBC studios and the U.S. Congress reinforces just how close we came to an unimaginable disaster [1].

Anthrax is a frightening pathogen, and the recent anthrax scare is eerily reminiscent of the near influenza pandemic that erupted in Hong Kong in 1997 where a renegade pathogenic avian influenza virus jumped directly from birds to humans [3]. Six of the 18 persons clinically diagnosed with this "bird flu" were dead within one week. If not for the weak infectivity of this particular influenza virus, the death toll from this outbreak could certainly have been far worse [4].

Besides illustrating our vulnerability to deadly microbes, is there a link between the anthrax and "bird flu" outbreaks? One link is furin, a cellular enzyme that activates a large number of molecules in secretory pathways. What is furin and how does it play a role in so many diseases? Furin is a type of enzyme known as a protease – a molecule that cuts larger proteins into smaller ones. But furin does not simply cut any protein. It cuts only the particular proteins that contain sites that are specifically recognized by furin. This type of furin-dependent cutting, or cleavage, creates a smaller, active protein product, and it is this active protein product that is responsible for the damage inflicted by pathogens. That is because pathogenic bacteria and viruses usurp the furin pathway to exert their virulence.

Research beginning in 1967 with the discovery of secretory pathway proteolysis led to the identification of furin in 1989 and eventually other members of the furin family, collectively known as proprotein convertases. However, furin is the most intensively studied member of this family, largely because of its demonstrated role in pathogenesis and disease.

Research by my laboratory and others during the last 12 years has revealed that furin is the cellular version of Dr. Jekyll and Mr. Hyde. On the one hand, furin plays an essential role in early embryogenesis and catalyzes the maturation of a diverse collection of proteins, ranging from growth factors and receptors to extracellular matrix proteins and even other proteases (reviewed in [5]). On the other hand, furin also has a decidedly dark side. For example, a number of bacterial toxins use furin as a catalyst to debilitate their victims. These toxins include the anthrax toxin and gangrene (that is, *Clostridium septicum* alpha-toxin), as well as one that burn victims and cystic fibrosis patients are susceptible to-- *Pseudomonas* exotoxin A [5]. Similarly, a number of pathogen viruses also absolutely require furin in order to be infectious—these include HIV, the virulent Hong Kong "bird flu", cytomegalovirus respiratory syncytial virus, and measles. Recent studies also suggest the virulence of Ebola is tightly coupled to the ability of this deadly virus to be processed by furin [6]. And furin also plays a role in devastating diseases such as cancer metastasis and rheumatoid arthritis [7-9].

In 1992, my laboratory collaborated with Dr. Steve Leppla at the NIH to report the characterization of furin's biochemical properties, including the identification of the site in precursor proteins that it recognizes and cuts [10]. Ironically, the anthrax toxin was the model we used to study furin-- or more precisely, we used a component of anthrax known as protective antigen. In these studies, we showed furin recognizes a site containing the amino acid sequence –Arg-X-

Lys/Arg-Arg$^{\downarrow}$- where Arg represents the amino acid arginine, Lys represents the amino acid lysine and X represents any amino acid. The arrow shows precisely where furin cuts the string of amino acids. We also showed that to perform its catalyzing function, furin at minimum requires the first and last arginines to form the sequence –Arg-X-X-Arg$^{\downarrow}$-. This identification proved crucial to our development of the first potent and selective furin inhibitor, summarized below.

Then, in a second paper published in collaboration with Dr. Leppla's group, we showed that furin is the cellular enzyme that activates the anthrax protective antigen – a step necessary for the deadly consequences of this toxin [11]. Protective antigen is released from *Bacillus anthracis* as a large, inactive protein that is cut by furin at the surface of cells to generate a smaller and active fragment of processed protective antigen—that is, its 63 kDa form. The 63 kDa protective antigen molecule binds to either of the two toxic factors also produced by the bacterium and delivers them into the cell, where they exert their virulent activities (reviewed in [12]). Subsequent studies by others have extended our findings with anthrax, to show that furin also catalyzes the activation of other deadly bacterial toxins, including *Pseudomonas* exotoxin A, shiga toxin, diphtheria toxin, proaerolysin, and the *Clostridium septicum* alpha-toxin [5].

What happens if you turn off or inactivate the furin enzyme? We showed that inactivation of furin by means of novel furin inhibitors will protect cells from being killed by *Pseudomonas* exotoxin A [13]. This finding suggests that furin might be a viable target for protection against many toxins. Because furin is required for the activation of anthrax protective antigen, we think furin is a viable target for research that may lead to effective therapies against anthrax.

The cleavage site specificity we discovered for furin using the anthrax toxin helped us and others to demonstrate a broad role for furin in viral pathogenesis. Many viruses express proteins that must be cut at furin sites (–Arg-X-Lys/Arg-Arg$^{\downarrow}$-) to generate infectious progeny. For example, we and others showed that the furin pathway is required for the production of many deadly viruses including the Hong Kong "bird flu", HIV, cytomegalovirus (a major complication for transplant patients and people suffering from AIDS), Measles virus and Respiratory syncytial virus [5]. For most of these viruses, furin is required for virus to fuse with target cells that will permit the virus to sustain itself. Furin is needed to process a protein on the outer surface of the viral envelope—if furin cuts the fusion protein correctly, the virus will be able to fuse with membranes on target cells, thus allowing the virus to spread. But we think that—based on our findings that turning off furin stops bacteria from reproducing--inhibitors of furin may also have an application as broad-based antiviral agents. In support of this, and as summarized below, we have found that inhibition of furin protects cells from a diverse set of viruses including HIV, human cytomegalovirus and measles.

Interestingly, the analysis of viral tropism – that is, the molecular determinants that enable a virus to spread throughout the body – shows that the virulence of many deadly viruses, including Ebola virus, is directly correlated with the ability of the virus to incorporate a consensus furin cleavage site within its envelope proteins. For example, the highly pathogenic Ebola Zaire and Ivory Coast strains, which cause fulminant hemorrhagic fever that kills 90% of the people who get it, contain a consensus furin site in the envelope proteins. But by contrast, the envelope protein of the relatively milder Ebola Reston strain lacks a consensus furin site and this isolate is not pathogenic to humans [14]. Similar compelling correlations are found with several other pathogenic viruses, and this may suggest that viruses mutate towards the furin pathway to become more deadly [15]. Thus, controlling furin activity may represent a biochemical block that the viruses cannot thwart.

Because so many diverse pathogenic bacteria and viruses rely on furin, it seems reasonable that creating furin inhibitors will yield a broad-based therapeutic. Studies by our laboratory and others suggest this is indeed possible. My laboratory used our knowledge of the requirements for cleavage of the anthrax protective antigen by furin to produce a potent and selective first generation furin inhibitor, called α_1-PDX [16]. α_1-PDX is a bioengineered variant of α_1-antitrypsin, which is a protease inhibitor found abundantly in blood. However, α_1-PDX contains the minimal consensus furin site—that is, -Arg-X-X-Arg$^{\downarrow}$-, which we determined with our anthrax studies. We have found this to be a highly selective and potent furin inhibitor [13]. Biochemical studies show α_1-PDX inhibits furin by acting as a "suicide substrate" – or a biochemical "mousetrap". It uses molecular chicanery to fool furin into attempting to cleave it. However, instead of releasing from furin, α_1-PDX remains covalently bound to the enzyme and causes furin to be eliminated from the cell. Thus, using α_1-PDX we can control the levels of cellular furin at will.

Does α_1-PDX protect cells from bacterial toxins and pathogenic viruses? Unequivocally, yes.

We reported that α_1-PDX protects cells from killing by *Pseudomonas* exotoxin A [13]. We also showed that α_1-PDX blocks the formation of infectious HIV-1, Measles virus and human cytomegalovirus [17, 18]. Thus, as hypothesized during our earlier studies, inhibition of furin can indeed lead to the creation of a broad-based anti-pathogen. To our knowledge, no other single strategy has yielded such broad success at blocking this collection of seemingly unrelated pathogens.

Remarkably, in addition to protecting against various microbial pathogens, very recent studies show inhibition of furin also holds promise to protect against debilitating diseases including cancer metastasis and arthritis. Several researchers have shown that furin initiates a cascade of reactions that eventually degrade tissue barriers and enable the tumor cells to metastasize and spread to different organs [9]. Moreover, several aggressive cancers are correlated with high levels of furin, supporting an important role for furin in tumor metastasis [8]. In collaboration with Dr. Andres Klein-Szanto at Fox Chase Cancer Center in Philadelphia, we showed α_1-PDX can shut down the furin cascade and block tumor metastasis in animal models [9]. The role of furin in arthritis is apparently due to its role in activating a factor called TGF-beta. TGF-beta cooperates with furin by activating enzymes that degrade cartilage in joints. Consistent with these findings, Dr. DuBois at the University of Sherbrooke, Quebec has recently found that treatment of animals with α_1-PDX lessens significantly the inflammation caused by arthritic injury (personal communication).

Clearly furin has a broad and important role in the activation of biological terrorist agents. It also contributes to the progression of debilitating human diseases. Together, these findings strongly suggest that furin is an excellent target for the generation of broad-based therapeutics. We are pleased that our invention of α_1-PDX has further illuminated the feasibility for this approach. Now, however, our task is to learn more about how to control furin levels in living organisms. We must also identify additional compounds and develop new chemistries that may ultimately yield potential drugs. The expertise of Drs. Smith and Balhorn in designing small molecule protease inhibitors will lead to development of these new compounds. Together, with the expertise of others at this hearing, we may indeed develop an exciting new strategy to protect against biological terrorist pathogens as well as debilitating human diseases.

References

1. *Update: Investigation of bioterrorism-related anthrax--Connecticut, 2001.* MMWR Morb Mortal Wkly Rep, 2001. **50**(48): p. 1077-9.
2. *From the Centers for Disease Control and Prevention. Update: investigation of bioterrorism-related Anthrax--Connecticut, 2001.* Jama, 2002. **287**(1): p. 34-5.
3. Subbarao, K., et al., *Characterization of an avian influenza A (H5N1) virus isolated from a child with a fatal respiratory illness.* Science, 1998. **279**(5349): p. 393-6.
4. Hatta, M., et al., *Molecular basis for high virulence of Hong Kong H5N1 influenza A viruses.* Science, 2001. **293**(5536): p. 1840-2.
5. Molloy, S.S., et al., *Bi-cycling the furin pathway: from TGN localization to pathogen activation and embryogenesis.* Trends Cell Biol, 1999. **9**(1): p. 28-35.
6. Volchkov, V.E., et al., *Processing of the Ebola virus glycoprotein by the proprotein convertase furin.* Proc Natl Acad Sci U S A, 1998. **95**(10): p. 5762-7.
7. Dubois, C.M., et al., *Evidence that furin is an authentic transforming growth factor-beta1-converting enzyme.* Am J Pathol, 2001. **158**(1): p. 305-16.
8. Bassi, D.E., et al., *Elevated furin expression in aggressive human head and neck tumors and tumor cell lines.* Mol Carcinog, 2001. **31**(4): p. 224-32.
9. Bassi, D.E., et al., *Furin inhibition results in absent or decreased invasiveness and tumorigenicity of human cancer cells.* Proc Natl Acad Sci U S A, 2001. **98**(18): p. 10326-31.
10. Molloy, S.S., et al., *Human furin is a calcium-dependent serine endoprotease that recognizes the sequence Arg-X-X-Arg and efficiently cleaves anthrax toxin protective antigen.* J Biol Chem, 1992. **267**(23): p. 16396-402.
11. Klimpel, K.R., et al., *Anthrax toxin protective antigen is activated by a cell surface protease with the sequence specificity and catalytic properties of furin.* Proc Natl Acad Sci U S A, 1992. **89**(21): p. 10277-81.
12. Duesbery, N.S. and G.F. Vande Woude, *Anthrax toxins.* Cell Mol Life Sci, 1999. **55**(12): p. 1599-609.
13. Jean, F., et al., *alpha1-Antitrypsin Portland, a bioengineered serpin highly selective for furin: application as an antipathogenic agent.* Proc Natl Acad Sci U S A, 1998. **95**(13): p. 7293-8.

14. Feldmann, H., et al., *The glycoproteins of Marburg and Ebola virus and their potential roles in pathogenesis.* Arch Virol Suppl, 1999. **15**: p. 159-69.

15. Rott, R., et al., *Influenza viruses, cell enzymes, and pathogenicity.* Am J Respir Crit Care Med, 1995. **152**(4 Pt 2): p. S16-9.

16. Anderson, E.D., et al., *Inhibition of HIV-1 gp160-dependent membrane fusion by a furin-directed alpha 1-antitrypsin variant.* J Biol Chem, 1993. **268**(33): p. 24887-91.

17. Watanabe, M., et al., *Engineered serine protease inhibitor prevents furin-catalyzed activation of the fusion glycoprotein and production of infectious measles virus.* J Virol, 1995. **69**(5): p. 3206-10.

18. Jean, F., et al., *A protein-based therapeutic for human cytomegalovirus infection.* Proc Natl Acad Sci U S A, 2000. **97**(6): p. 2864-9.

7

Mr. BURTON. Thank you, Doctor.

Those buzzers you heard going off in the middle of your testimony indicate there's a vote on the floor of the House. So we will recess and come back here in about 10 minutes, and then we'll go to Dr. Collier and Dr. Young. Then we'll get to questions. So please bear with us. We'll be back in about 10 minutes.

[Recess.]

Mr. BURTON. If we can get everybody back to the witness table, we'll restart the hearing and there will be Members wandering back in.

Dr. Young, I understand it's your birthday today. Do you want me to sing to you "Happy birthday"? [Laughter.]

It's your 29th, is it? [Laughter.]

Well, you look very young, anyhow. Happy birthday to you.

Our next panelist is Dr. Collier. Dr. Collier is a professor of microbiology and molecular genetics at Harvard Medical School. Harvard, I've heard of that school. That's part of the Ivy League, isn't it?

You're recognized, Dr. Collier.

Mr. COLLIER. It's an honor to be here to testify today.

My career has largely been devoted to research on bacterial toxins, focusing on their structures of and how they damage cells of the body. For the past 15 years we have devoted considerable effort to understanding the structure and action of anthrax toxin. Our work, together with that of many others, including Steve Leppla, Art Friedlander, John Young, Bob Littington, and others, has given an increasingly detailed understanding of this toxin and how it acts. This, in turn, has revealed new ways to inhibit the action; that is, new types of anti-toxins, new approaches to making anti-toxins.

I'll just briefly describe in just a few minutes two new ways, two new types of anti-toxins that have emerged directly from our understanding of the structure and action of this toxin. Then I'll make brief comments about our experiences in trying to identify a path to develop these new anti-toxins into therapeutic reagents.

These anti-toxins, a third one that was developed in collaboration with John Young, and that Dr. Young will describe, are described in an article coauthored by the two of us in the March issue of Scientific American. Hopefully, you received copies of this.

So, as you have heard, the anthrax toxin consists of three proteins that the anthrax bacterium releases into its environment. None of these three proteins alone is toxic, but they act together to cause damage to our cells. Two of the proteins, called lethal factor and edema factor, are enzymes that act inside our cells to alter certain aspects of metabolism. Alone these factors are unable to penetrate the protective membrane barrier that surrounds our cells. Therefore, they cannot enter. Therefore, they're not toxic by themselves.

This is where the third protein comes into play. This is the protein called protective antigen [PA]. This protein assembles on the surface of our cells into what can be thought of as a molecular syringe that is able to inject the other two proteins into the cell, figuratively speaking. Once inside the cell, the edema factor and lethal factor have access then to their molecular targets. They modify these, and that disrupts metabolism in ways that ultimately lead to death of the human.

So figure 1 illustrates the steps by which the syringe assembles and acts. I've only shown here the bare essentials of this process to keep it simple. If you'll refer to the Scientific American article later, you'll see that there's some complexities that I've left out.

But, as shown, the first step is on the left here, the PA molecular released by the bacterium binds to its receptor, ATR, that Dr. Young will describe in greater detail. There are about 10,000 or more copies of the receptor for PA on an average cell. Thus, you can get up to about that many copies of PA bound to a cell.

Once they're bound, they are activated by a member of the furin class of proteases that have been described, and then they come together in clusters of seven. We've distributed for you these little molecular models of the molecular syringe, as it were, the group of seven of these heptamers. These were generated by Dr. Timothy Herman at the Milwaukee School of Engineering and provided to us today for this hearing.

So, once the syringe is generated by aggregation of these single molecules of activated PA, it's then loaded with its cargo, EF and LF. That's shown, I think, as the next-to-the-last step there, where we've only shown LF, the red molecule there on the screen coming down and binding to the surface of the heptamer. The syringe is now loaded. The final step then is for the syringe to inject the EF and LF into the cytosol. There it acts to generate the effects that will ultimately lead to death.

So let me now, with that background then, proceed to describe the two new concepts about anti-toxins. Figure 2 shows the first one. This is the concept of a dominant negative inhibitor [DNI]. The DNI consists of a mutated form of the PA molecule. So PA molecule consists of a long string of amino acids, some 700 or so amino acids.

We have found certain places in that long string of amino acids where we can change just one or two amino acids, totally change the properties of this molecule. The dominant negative inhibitor will still—it will combine with the normal PA that's produced by the bacteria in the body, but generate a mixed heptamer. This is illustrated here on the model. So the white one is meant to be a dominant negative inhibitor.

If you now have one copy of the dominant negative inhibitor—we think one copy is enough—one copy incorporated into the heptamer, the syringe won't plunge. It will still bind the EF and LF, and so you will get a complex, but the complex is totally inactive.

So this is one potential way—this has been shown to work in animals as well as in cell culture—to block toxin action. So this is one way, then, that we think needs to be explored as a possible route to a new type of anti-toxin, the dominant negative inhibitor.

The next slide shows the second approach that I wanted to illustrate and that I wanted to tell you about and is figure 3. This is a type of anti-toxin that was developed, it's a synthetic anti-toxin developed through organic chemistry, developed in collaboration with George Whitesides, a professor in the Chemistry Department at Harvard. It's a synthetic so-called polyvalent inhibitor that blocks loading of the syringe with its cargo.

So we first isolated a peptide that's at the upper right here that would weakly block the interaction of the EF and LF with the syringe, and, thus, block those binding sites. Then we grafted many copies of that peptide inhibitor onto a flexible backbone, giving you then a polyvalental inhibitor that can sit down now on this seven-membered syringe, and you have many interaction points then. You can block essentially all seven sites with the polyvalent inhibitor. So this is another approach that's been explored. As I said, Dr. Young will describe the third one that we've been involved with.

I want to emphasize at this point that all of the research that I've described that I've performed actually in my career, almost all the research has been done under grants from the National Institute of Allergy and Infectious Disease. The system of peer-reviewed grants that the NIH uses is, in my view, an outstanding system that's served the Nation well as a vehicle for building high-quality knowledge base that's needed to develop new treatments for diseases of mankind. It accomplishes this with a minimum of bureaucracy.

This brings us to the question, then, of how to accelerate research and development of new therapeutics against anthrax. When we first discovered the strong anti-toxin activity of the dominant negative inhibitors, now over a year ago and long before the anthrax attacks of last fall, we began exploring ways to do the translational research needed to develop them into clinically useful drugs. These agents were ready to be developed in a corporate setting. The university setting is not appropriate for this type of research, and the research would be expensive because of the containment conditions required, among other things, the large number of animal experiments required. If the product proved efficacious, there would be only one customer, the Federal Government.

It was clear, then, from the outset that the developmental research would need to be done under some form of government/corporate partnership. Possible scenarios were discussed with various agencies, but a rapid path has been illusive until recently, when DARPA became interested in the project. It appears likely now that funds and the managerial partnership necessary to conduct this research on a fast track will now be forthcoming from DARPA.

USAMRIID has been helpful also and will be contributing, we expect, funds to the project as well. So we hope to learn through research on animal models of infectious anthrax, conducted within the shortest possible time, whether or not the dominant negative inhibitors and the polyvalent inhibitors will be truly efficacious in treating anthrax in an infected animal model because experiments have not been done yet.

From our experience to date, it appears that the DARPA model may be worth considering by other agencies that are seeking to support the developmental phase of studies to generate countermeasures against biological agents of terrorism.

Apart from this, another major barrier to development of such countermeasures is the dearth of high-level containment facilities for testing new therapeutic agents in animal infection models, a major problem. Rectifying this serious and widely recognized impediment would greatly accelerate progress in this area.

Thank you.

[The prepared statement of Mr. Collier follows:]

Testimony to be presented before the House Committee on Government Reform on "Quickening the Pace of Research in Protecting Against Anthrax and Other Biological Terrorist Agents-A Look at Toxin Interference"

My career has largely been devoted to research on bacterial toxins, focusing on their structures of and how they damage cells of the body. For the past 15 years we have devoted considerable effort to the study of anthrax toxin. Our work, together with that of Steve Leppla, Art Friedlander, John Young and others, has given an increasingly detailed understanding of how anthrax toxin acts. This in turn has revealed new ways to inhibit its action—that is, new types of antitoxins. I shall briefly describe two new types of antitoxins that we have developed and then make brief comments about our experiences in identifying a path to develop them into useful therapeutic agents. (These antitoxins and a third, developed in collaboration with John Young, are described in an article coauthored by the two of us in the March issue of *Scientific American*.)

The anthrax toxin consists of three proteins that the anthrax bacterium releases into its environment. None of the three proteins alone is toxic; rather, they act together to cause damage. Two of the proteins, called Lethal Factor (LF) and Edema Factor (EF), are enzymes that act inside our cells to alter aspects of metabolism. Alone, however, these Factors cannot penetrate the protective membrane barrier that surrounds the cell. This is where the third component of the toxin comes into play. This protein, called Protective Antigen (or PA), assembles into what can be thought of as a "molecular syringe" that injects the Lethal and Edema Factors across the membrane and into the cell interior. Once inside the cell, these Factors have access to their molecular targets and disrupt metabolism in ways that lead to death of the victim.

Figure 1 illustrates the steps by which the syringe assembles and acts. (Only the bare essentials of this process are shown in the figure, to avoid confusion; refer to the *Scientific American* article for greater detail.) As shown, PA first binds to its receptor, ATR. There are 10,000 or more copies of the receptor on the average cell; thus up to that many copies of PA can bind. These receptor-bound PA molecules then are activated by a member of the furin family of proteases (a step not shown) and then come together in clusters of 7. This heptamer of PA represents the syringe. Next the syringe is loaded with its cargo, LF or EF. Finally the syringe punctures the membrane and injects LF and EF (the endocytosis step preceding injection has been omitted from the figure.)

Figure 2 illustrates the concept underlying one of our antitoxins. The so-called Dominant-Negative Inhibitor (DNI) consists of a mutated form of the PA molecule that is able to perform all of the tasks performed by normal PA, except the last step: the njection of LF or EF into the cell. More importantly, DNI combines with normal PA on the cell to create mixed heptamers that are defective in injection. In effect, the DNI tricks the normal PA molecules into thinking it is one of their own, and once included, it blocks the injection mechanism.

Figure 3 illustrates the concept underlying the second of our antitoxins, which was developed in collaboration with the group of George Whitesides (Chemistry Department, Harvard). It is a synthetic, polyvalent inhibitor (PVI) that blocks loading of the syringe with its cargo (LF and EF). We first isolated a peptide that weakly inhibits interaction of LF and EF with their binding sites on PA and then grafted many copies of it onto a flexible carrier molecule, creating the PVI. The grafted peptides on a PVI molecule can bind to multiple sites on the PA heptamer (up to seven), causing strong binding and thus strong inhibition of EF and LF binding. Both the DNI and the PVI have been shown to block toxin action in a rat model system, and we think they represent promising approaches to therapy of anthrax (for use in conjunction with antibiotics.)

Let me emphasize at this point that all of the research described has been performed under grants from the National Institute of Allergy and Infectious Diseases. The system of peer reviewed grants has served the nation well as a vehicle for building a high-quality knowledge base needed to develop new treatments for diseases of mankind; and it accomplishes this with a minimum of beaurocracy.

This brings us to the question of how to accelerate research and development of new therapeutics against anthrax. When we first discovered the strong antitoxin activity of DNIs, now over a year ago ago and long before the anthrax attacks of last fall, we began exploring ways to do the translational research needed to develop them into clinically useful drugs. These agents were ready to be developed in a corporate setting; the university setting was not appropriate for the type of research that needed to be done. The research would be expensive, because of the containment conditions required, and if the product proved efficacious there would be only one customer: the federal government. It was thus clear from the outset that the developmental research would need to be done under some form of government-corporate partnership.

Possible scenarios were discussed with various agencies, but a rapid path was elusive until recently, when DARPA became interested in the project. It appears likely now that the funds and managerial partnership necessary to conduct this research on a fast track will now be forthcoming from DARPA. USAMRIID has been helpful and will also be contributing funds to the project. We hope to learn through research on animal models of infectious anthrax, conducted within the shortest possible time, whether or not the DNIs will be truly efficacious in treating anthrax. From our experience to date, it appears that the DARPA model may be worth considering by other agencies seeking to support the development phase of studies to generate countermeasures against biological agents of terrorism.

Apart from this, another major barrier to development of such countermeasures is the dearth of high-level containment facilities for testing of new therapeutic agents in animal infection models. Rectifying this serious and widely recognized impediment would accelerate progress in this area.

Respectrully submitted,

R. John Collier, Ph.D.
Professor, Harvard Medical School

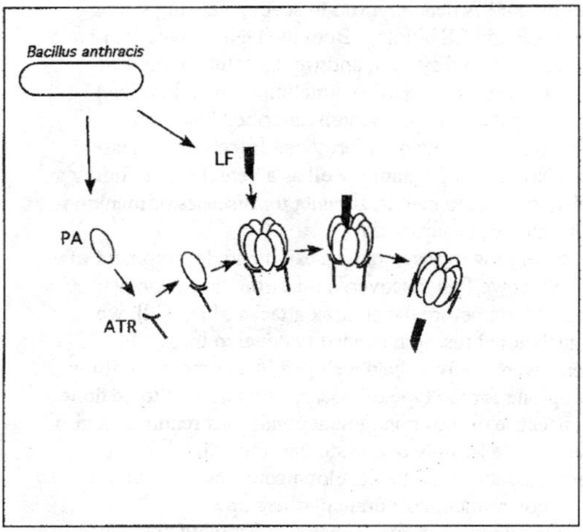

Figure 1: Assembly of the PA heptamer (the "molecular syringe") at the mammalian cell surface, "charging" of the syringe with LF, its "cargo", and translocation of LF into the cell.

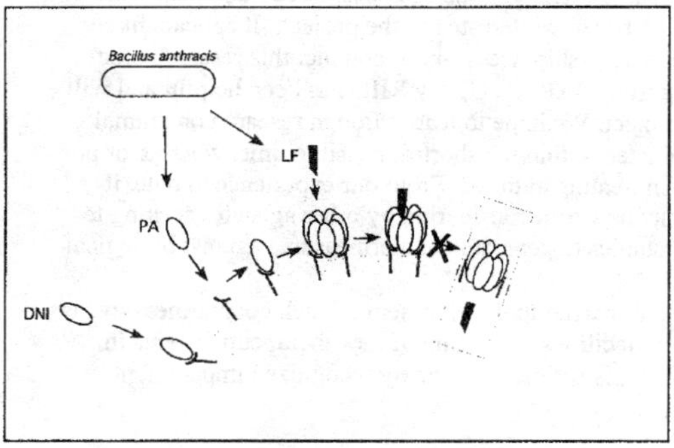

Figure 2: Incorporation of DNI into PA heptamer during self-assembly process, blocking the membrane translocation step of toxin action. (Based on the findings of Sellman, Mourez, and Collier, *Science* 292:695-697 2001)

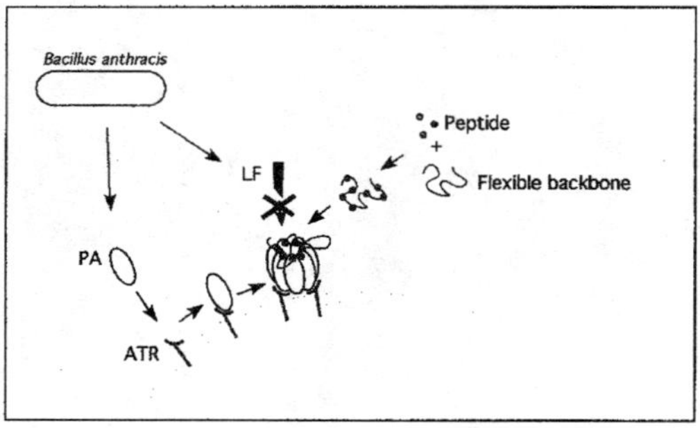

Figure 3: Action of PVI to block binding of LF to the PA heptamer. EF binding is blocked in the same way. (Based on the findings of Mourez et al., *Nature Biotechnology* 19:958-961 2001)

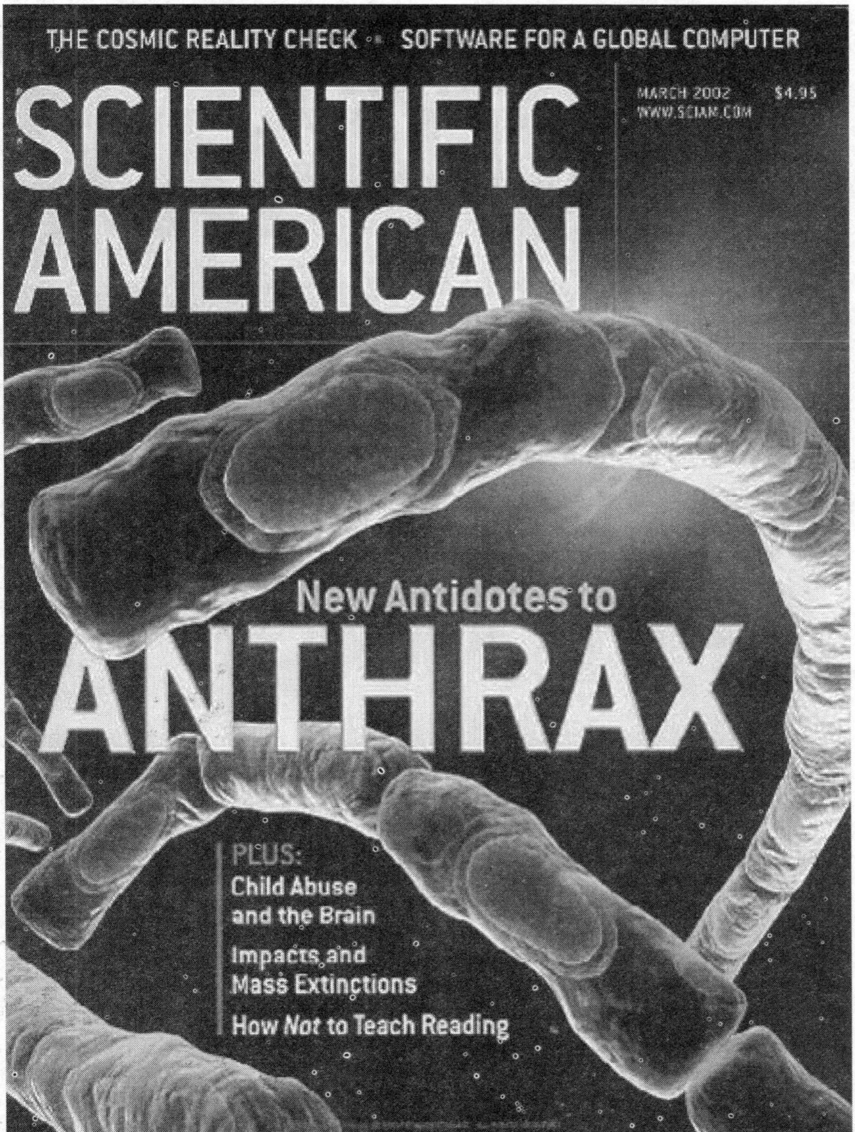
THE COSMIC REALITY CHECK • SOFTWARE FOR A GLOBAL COMPUTER
SCIENTIFIC AMERICAN
MARCH 2002 $4.95
WWW.SCIAM.COM
New Antidotes to
ANTHRAX
PLUS:
Child Abuse and the Brain
Impacts and Mass Extinctions
How Not to Teach Reading

ATTACKING ANTHRAX

Recent discoveries are suggesting much-needed strategies for improving prevention and treatment. High on the list: ways to neutralize the anthrax bacterium's fiendish toxin

by John A. T. Young and R. John Collier

CULTURES OF CELLS survived exposure to the anthrax toxin after being treated with a potential antitoxin. Michael Mourez of Harvard University holds a plate containing the cultures.

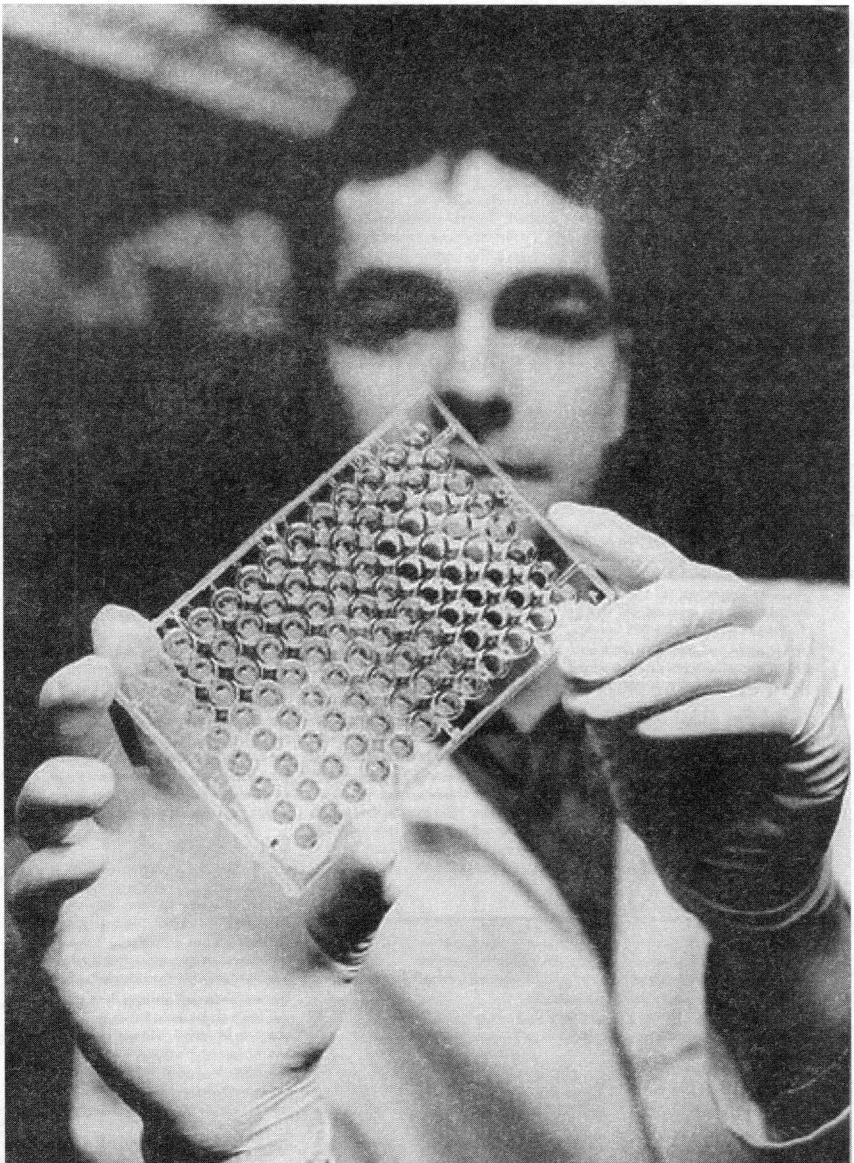

The need for new anthrax therapies became all too clear last fall

when five people died of inhalation anthrax, victims of the first purposeful release of anthrax spores in the U.S. Within days of showing initially unalarming symptoms, the patients were gone, despite intensive treatment with antibiotics. Six others became seriously ill as well before pulling through.

Fortunately, our laboratories and others began studying the causative bacterium, *Bacillus anthracis,* and seeking antidotes long before fall 2001. Recent findings are now pointing the way to novel medicines and improved vaccines. Indeed, in the past year alone, the two of us and our collaborators have reported on three promising drug prototypes.

An Elusive Killer

THE NEW IDEAS for fighting anthrax have emerged from ongoing research into how *B. anthracis* causes disease and death. Anthrax does not spread from individual to individual. A person (or animal) gets sick only after incredibly hardy spores enter the body through a cut in the skin, through contaminated food or through spore-laden air. Inside the body the spores molt into "vegetative," or actively dividing, cells.

Anthrax bacteria that colonize the skin or digestive tract initially do damage locally and may cause self-limited ailments: black sores and swelling in the first instance; possibly vomiting and abdominal pain and bleeding in the second. If bacterial growth persists unchecked in the skin or gastrointestinal tract, however, the microbes may eventually invade the bloodstream and thereby cause systemic disease.

Inhaled spores that reach deep into the lungs tend to waste little time where they land. They typically convert to the vegetative form and travel quickly to lymph nodes in the middle of the chest, where many of the cells find ready access to the blood. (Meanwhile bacteria that remain in the chest set the stage for a breath-robbing buildup of fluid around the lungs.)

Extensive replication in the blood is generally what kills patients who succumb to anthrax. *B. anthracis*'s ability to expand so successfully derives from its secretion of two substances, known as virulence factors, that can profoundly derail the immune defenses meant to keep bacterial growth in check. One of these factors encases the vegetative cells in a polymer capsule that inhibits ingestion by the immune system's macrophages and neutrophils—the scavenger cells that normally degrade disease-causing bacteria. The capsule's partner in crime is an extraordinary toxin that works its way into those scavenger cells, or phagocytes, and interferes with their usual bacteria-killing actions.

The anthrax toxin, which also enters other cells, is thought to contribute to mortal illness not only by dampening immune responses but also by playing a direct role. Evidence for this view includes the observation that the toxin alone, in the absence of bacteria, can kill animals. Conversely, inducing the immune system to neutralize the toxin prevents *B. anthracis* from causing disease.

A Terrible Toxin

HARRY SMITH and his co-workers at the Microbiological Research Establishment in Wiltshire, England, discovered the toxin in the 1950s. Aware of its central part in anthrax's lethality, many researchers have since focused on learning how the substance "intoxicates" cells—gets into them and disrupts their activities. Such details offer essential clues to blocking its effects. Stephen H. Leppla and Arthur M. Friedlander, while at the U.S. Army Medical Research Institute of Infectious Diseases, initiated that effort with their colleagues in the 1980s; the two

Overview/*Anthrax*

- A three-part toxin produced by the anthrax bacterium, *Bacillus anthracis,* contributes profoundly to the symptoms and lethality of anthrax.
- The toxin causes trouble only when it gets into the cytosol of cells, the material that bathes the cell's internal compartments.
- Drugs that prevented the toxin from reaching the cytosol would probably go a long way toward limiting illness and saving the lives of people infected by the anthrax bacterium.
- Analyses of how the toxin enters cells have recently led to the discovery of several potential antitoxins.

JASON GROW (preceding page)

Detecting Anthrax

Rapid sensing would save lives

By Rocco Casagrande

IF A TERRORIST GROUP spread anthrax spores into the open air, the release could affect large numbers of people but would probably go unnoticed until victims showed up at hospitals. Many would undoubtedly seek help too late to be saved by current therapies. Much illness could be prevented, however, if future defenses against anthrax attacks included sensors that raised an alarm soon after spores appeared in the environment. The needed instruments are not yet ready for deployment, but various designs that incorporate cutting-edge technology are being developed.

Environmental sensors must discriminate between disease-causing agents (pathogens) and the thousands of similar but harmless microorganisms that colonize air, water and soil. Most of the tools being investigated work by detecting unique molecules on the surface of the pathogens of interest or by picking out stretches of DNA found only in those organisms.

The Canary, which is being developed at the Massachusetts Institute of Technology Lincoln Laboratory, is an innovative example of the devices that detect pathogens based on unique surface molecules. The sensors of the Canary consist of living cells—B cells of the immune system—that have been genetically altered to emit light when their calcium levels change. Protruding from these cells are receptors that will bind only to a unique part of a surface molecule on a particular pathogen. When the cells in the sensor bind to their target, that binding triggers the release of calcium ions from stores within the cells, which in turn causes the cells to give off light. The Canary can discern more than one type of pathogen by running a sample through several cell-filled modules, each of which reacts to a selected microorganism.

The GeneXpert system, developed by Cepheid, in Sunnyvale, Calif., is an example of a gene-centered approach. It begins its work by extracting DNA from microorganisms in a sample. Then, if a pathogen of concern is present, small primers (strips of genetic material able to recognize specific short sequences of DNA) latch onto the ends of DNA fragments unique to the pathogen. Next, through a procedure called the polymerase chain reaction (PCR), the system makes many copies of the bound DNA, adding fluorescent labels to the new copies along the way. Within about 30 minutes GeneXpert can make enough DNA to reveal whether even a small amount of the worrisome organism inhabited the original sample.

This system contains multiple PCR reaction chambers with distinct primer sets to allow the detection of different pathogens simultaneously. Furthermore, the GeneXpert system could be used to determine whether the anthrax bacterium is present in a nasal swab taken from a patient in as little as half an hour, significantly faster than the time it takes for conventional microbiological techniques to yield results.

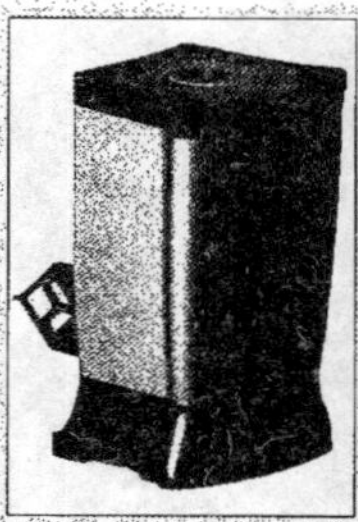

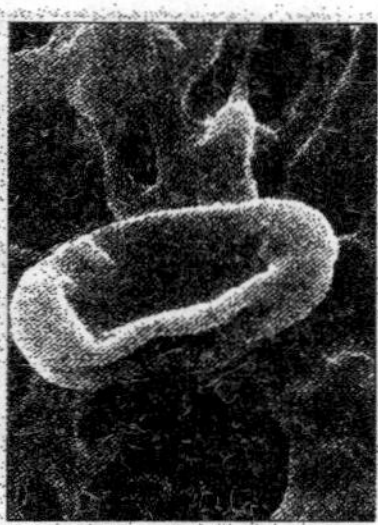

CARTRIDGE used in the experimental GeneXpert system is about as tall as an adult's thumb (*left*). Inside, sound waves bombard material to be tested, causing any cells to break open and release their DNA. If a pathogen of interest is present, its DNA will be amplified in the arrow-shaped reaction tube (*protrusion*), and the edges of the arrowhead will fluoresce. The micrograph (*right*) shows the remains of a cell that has disgorged its contents.

Instruments designed specifically to detect spores of the anthrax bacterium or of closely related microbes (such as the one that causes botulism) can exploit the fact that such spores are packed full of dipicolinic acid (DPA)—a compound, rarely found elsewhere in nature, that helps them to survive harsh environmental conditions. Molecules that fluoresce when bound to DPA have shown promise in chemically based anthrax detectors. "Electronic noses," such as the Cyranose detection system made by Cyrano Sciences in Pasadena, Calif., could possibly "smell" the presence of DPA in an air sample laced with anthrax spores.

The true danger of an anthrax release lies in its secrecy. If an attack is discovered soon after it occurs and if exposed individuals receive treatment promptly, victims have an excellent chance of surviving. By enhancing early detection, sensors based on the systems discussed above or on entirely different technologies could effectively remove a horrible weapon from a terrorist's arsenal.

ROCCO CASAGRANDE is a scientist at Surface Logix in Brighton, Mass., where he is developing methods and devices for detecting biological weapons.

of us and others took up the task somewhat later.

The anthrax toxin turns out to consist of three proteins, named protective antigen, edema factor and lethal factor. These components cooperate but are not always joined together physically. They are harmless individually until they attach to and enter cells, which they accomplish in a highly orchestrated fashion.

First, protective antigen binds to the surface of a cell, where an enzyme trims off its outermost tip. Next, seven of those trimmed molecules combine to form a ring-shaped structure, or heptamer, that captures the two factors and is transported to an internal membrane-bound compartment called an endosome. Mild acidity in this compartment causes the heptamer to change shape in a way that leads to the transport of edema factor and lethal factor across the endosomal membrane into the cytosol (the internal matrix of cells), where they do their mischief. In essence, the heptamer is like a syringe loaded with edema factor and lethal factor, and the slight acidity of the endosome causes the

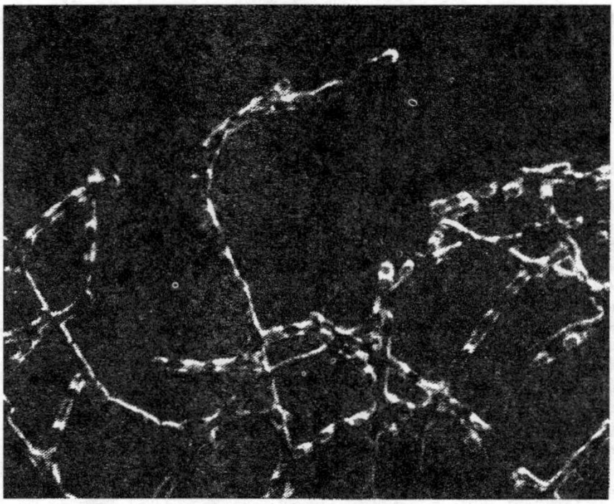

ACTIVELY DIVIDING CELLS of the anthrax bacterium arrange themselves into chains that resemble linked boxcars.

syringe to pierce the membrane of the endosome and inject the toxic factors into the cytosol.

Edema factor and lethal factor catalyze different molecular reactions in cells. Edema factor upsets the controls on ion and water flow across cell membranes and thereby promotes the swelling of tissues. In phagocytes, it also saps energy that would otherwise be used to engulf bacteria.

The precise behavior of lethal factor, which could be more important in causing patient deaths, is less clear. Scientists do know that it is a protease (a protein-cutting enzyme) and that it cleaves enzymes in a family known as MAPKKs. Now they are trying to tease out the molecular events that follow such cleavage and to uncover the factor's specific contributions to disease and death.

THE AUTHORS

JOHN A. T. YOUNG and *R. JOHN COLLIER* have collaborated for several years on investigating the anthrax toxin. Young is Howard M. Temin Professor of Cancer Research in the McArdle Laboratory for Cancer Research at the University of Wisconsin–Madison. Collier, who has studied anthrax for more than 14 years, is Maude and Lillian Presley Professor of Microbiology and Molecular Genetics at Harvard Medical School.

Therapeutic Tactics

CERTAINLY DRUGS able to neutralize the anthrax toxin would help the immune system fight bacterial multiplication and would probably reduce a patient's risk of dying. At the moment, antibiotics given to victims of inhalation anthrax may control microbial expansion but leave the toxin free to wreak havoc.

In principle, toxin activity could be halted by interfering with any of the steps in the intoxication process. An attractive approach would stop the sequence almost before it starts, by preventing protective antigen from attaching to cells. Scientists realized almost 10 years ago that this protein initiated toxin entry by binding to some specific protein on the surface of cells; when cells were treated with enzymes that removed all their surface proteins, protective antigen found no footing. Until very recently, though, no one knew which of the countless proteins on cells served as the crucial receptor.

The two of us, with our colleagues Kenneth Bradley, Jeremy Mogridge and Michael Mourez, found the receptor last summer. Detailed analysis of this molecule (now named ATR, for anthrax toxin receptor) then revealed that it spans the cell membrane and protrudes from it. The protruding part contains an area resembling a region that serves in other receptors as an attachment site for particular proteins. This discovery suggested that the area was the place where protective antigen latched onto ATR, and indeed it is.

We have not yet learned the normal function of the receptor, which surely did not evolve specifically to allow the anthrax toxin into cells. Nevertheless, knowledge of the molecule's makeup is enabling us to begin testing inhibitors of its activity. We have had success, for instance, with a compound called sATR, which is a soluble form of the receptor domain that binds to protective antigen. When sATR molecules are mixed into the medium surrounding cells, they serve as effective decoys, tricking protective antigen into binding to them instead of to its true receptor on cells.

We are now trying to produce sATR in the amounts needed for evaluating its ability to combat anthrax in rodents and nonhuman primates—experiments that must be done before any new drug can be considered for fighting anthrax in people. Other groups are examining whether carefully engineered antibodies (highly specific molecules of the immune system) might bind tightly to protective antigen in ways that will keep it from coupling with its receptor.

More Targets

SCIENTISTS ARE ALSO seeking ways to forestall later steps in the intoxication pathway. For example, a team from Harvard has constructed a drug able to clog the regions of the heptamer that grasp edema and lethal factors. The group—from the laboratories of one of us (Collier) and George M. Whitesides—reasoned that a plugged heptamer would be unable to draw the factors into cells.

We began by screening randomly constructed peptides (short chains of amino acids) to see if any of them bound to the

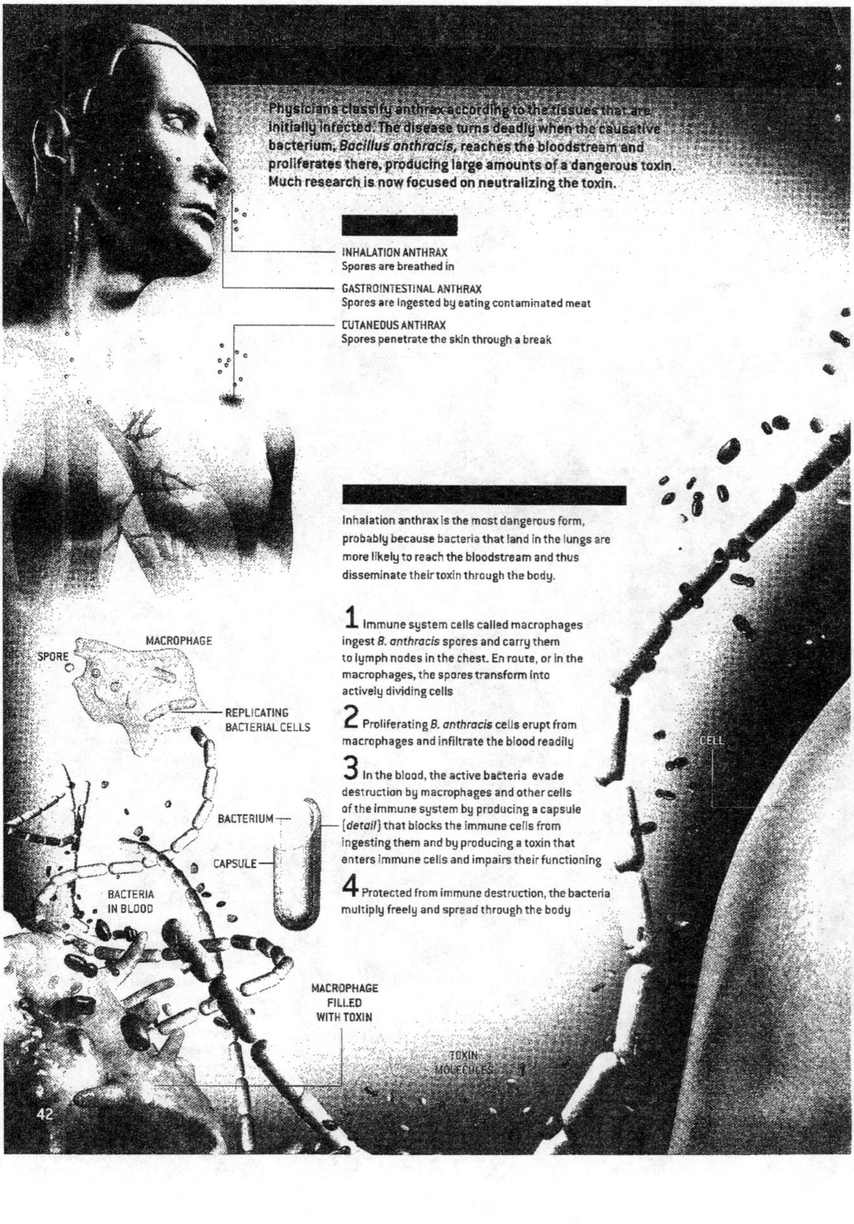
Physicians classify anthrax according to the tissues that are initially infected. The disease turns deadly when the causative bacterium, *Bacillus anthracis*, reaches the bloodstream and proliferates there, producing large amounts of a dangerous toxin. Much research is now focused on neutralizing the toxin.

INHALATION ANTHRAX
Spores are breathed in

GASTROINTESTINAL ANTHRAX
Spores are ingested by eating contaminated meat

CUTANEOUS ANTHRAX
Spores penetrate the skin through a break

Inhalation anthrax is the most dangerous form, probably because bacteria that land in the lungs are more likely to reach the bloodstream and thus disseminate their toxin through the body.

1 Immune system cells called macrophages ingest *B. anthracis* spores and carry them to lymph nodes in the chest. En route, or in the macrophages, the spores transform into actively dividing cells

2 Proliferating *B. anthracis* cells erupt from macrophages and infiltrate the blood readily

3 In the blood, the active bacteria evade destruction by macrophages and other cells of the immune system by producing a capsule (*detail*) that blocks the immune cells from ingesting them and by producing a toxin that enters immune cells and impairs their functioning

4 Protected from immune destruction, the bacteria multiply freely and spread through the body

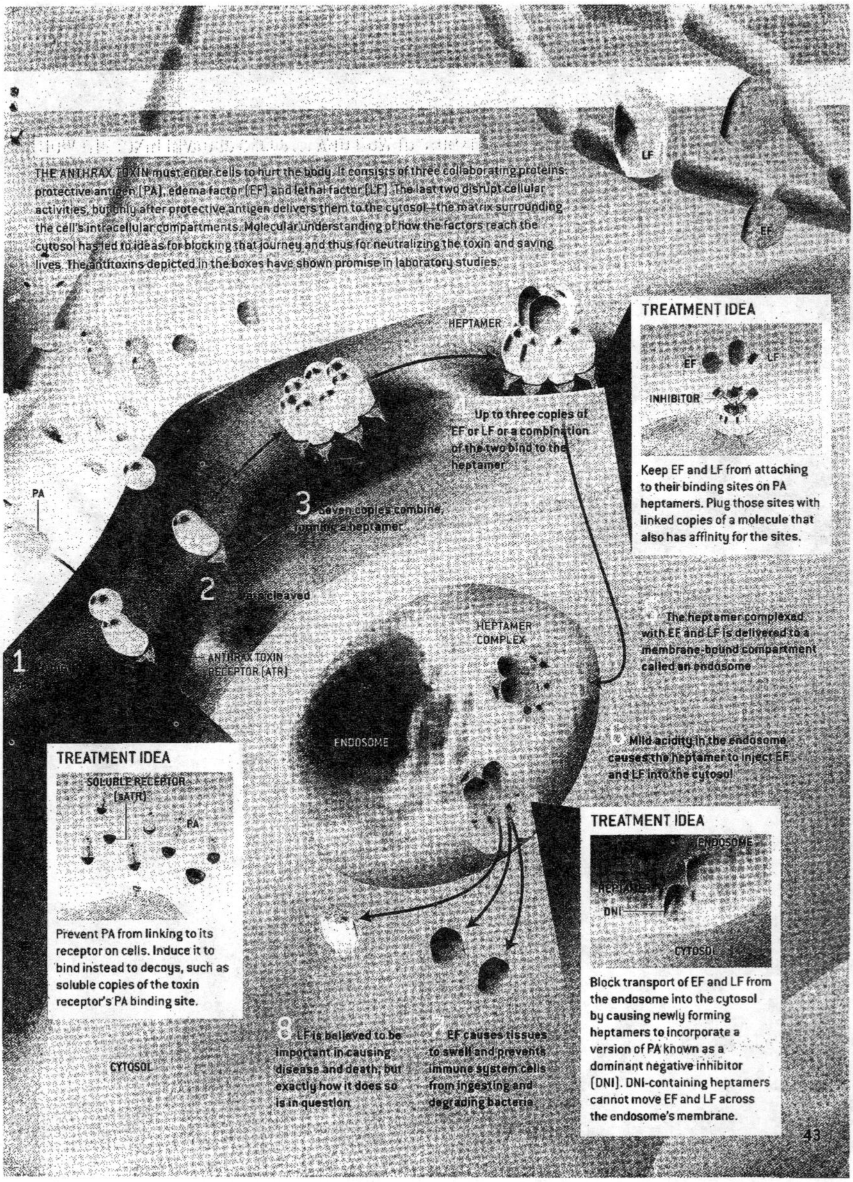
THE ANTHRAX TOXIN must enter cells to hurt the body. It consists of three collaborating proteins: protective antigen (PA), edema factor (EF) and lethal factor (LF). The last two disrupt cellular activities, but only after protective antigen delivers them to the cytosol—the matrix surrounding the cell's intracellular compartments. Molecular understanding of how the factors reach the cytosol has led to ideas for blocking that journey and thus for neutralizing the toxin and saving lives. The antitoxins depicted in the boxes have shown promise in laboratory studies.
LF
EF
PA
1
ANTHRAX TOXIN RECEPTOR (ATR)
2
3 Seven copies combine, forming a heptamer
HEPTAMER
Up to three copies of EF or LF or a combination of the two bind to the heptamer
TREATMENT IDEA
EF
LF
INHIBITOR
Keep EF and LF from attaching to their binding sites on PA heptamers. Plug those sites with linked copies of a molecule that also has affinity for the sites.
The heptamer complexed with EF and LF is delivered to a membrane-bound compartment called an endosome
HEPTAMER COMPLEX
ENDOSOME
Mild acidity in the endosome causes the heptamer to inject EF and LF into the cytosol
TREATMENT IDEA
SOLUBLE RECEPTOR (sATR)
PA
Prevent PA from linking to its receptor on cells. Induce it to bind instead to decoys, such as soluble copies of the toxin receptor's PA binding site.
TREATMENT IDEA
ENDOSOME
DNI
CYTOSOL
Block transport of EF and LF from the endosome into the cytosol by causing newly forming heptamers to incorporate a version of PA known as a dominant negative inhibitor (DNI). DNI-containing heptamers cannot move EF and LF across the endosome's membrane.
CYTOSOL
8 LF is believed to be important in causing disease and death, but exactly how it does so is in question
EF causes tissues to swell and prevents immune system cells from ingesting and degrading bacteria
43

heptamer. One did, so we examined its ability to block toxin activity. It worked, but weakly. Assuming that fitting many plugs into the heptamer's binding domains for edema and lethal factor would be more effective, we took advantage of chemical procedures devised by Whitesides's group and linked an average of 22 copies of the peptide to a flexible polymer. That construction showed itself to be a strong inhibitor of toxin action—more than 7,000 times better than the free peptide—both in cell cultures and in rats.

Another exciting agent, and the one probably closest to human testing, would alter the heptamer itself. This compound was discovered after Bret R. Sellman in Collier's group noted that when certain mutant forms of protective antigen were mixed with normal forms, the heptamers formed on cells as usual but were unable to inject edema and lethal factors into the cytosol. Remarkably, some of these mutants were so disruptive that a single copy in a heptamer completely prevented injection.

In a study reported last April, these mutants—known as dominant negative inhibitors, or DNIs—proved to be potent blockers of the anthrax toxin in cell cultures and in rats. Relatively small amounts of selected DNIs neutralized an amount of protective antigen and lethal factor that would otherwise kill a rat in 90 minutes. These findings suggest that each mutant copy of protective antigen is capable of inactivating six normal copies in the bloodstream and that it would probably reduce toxin activity in patients dramatically.

Of course, as more and more questions about the toxin are answered, scientists should discover further treatment ideas. Now that the receptor for protective antigen has been identified, researchers can use it as a target in screening tests aimed at finding drugs able to bar the receptor from binding to protective antigen. And understanding of the receptor's three-dimensional structure would reveal the precise contact points between protective antigen and the receptor, enabling drugmakers to custom-design receptor blocking agents.

Scientists would also like to uncover the molecular interactions that enable protective antigen heptamers to move from the cell surface into endosomes inside the cell. Impeding that migration should be very useful. And what happens after lethal factor cleaves MAPKK enzymes? How do those subsequent events affect cells? Although the latter question remains a vexing challenge, recent study of lethal factor has brightened the prospects for finding drugs able to inactivate it. Last November, Robert C. Liddington of the Burnham Institute in La Jolla, Calif., and his colleagues in several laboratories published the three-dimensional structure of the part of lethal factor that acts on MAPKK molecules. That site can now become a target for drug screening or design.

New leads for drugs should also emerge from the recent sequencing of the code letters composing the *B. anthracis* genome. By finding genes that resemble those of known functions in other organisms, biologists are likely to discover additional information about how the anthrax bacterium causes disease and how to stop it.

The continuing research should yield several antitoxins. To be most effective, such drugs will probably be used with antibiotics, much as cocktails of antiviral drugs are recommended for treating HIV infection.

To be most effective, antitoxins will probably be USED WITH ANTIBIOTICS, much as cocktails of antiviral drugs are recommended for treating HIV infection.

Promising Preventives

AS PLANS TO IMPROVE therapies proceed, so does work on better vaccines. Vaccines against toxin-producing bacteria often prime the immune system to neutralize the toxin of concern as soon as it appears in the body, thus preventing disease. Livestock in parts of the U.S. receive preparations consisting of *B. anthracis* cells that lack the protective capsule and thus replicate poorly. A similar vaccine for humans has been used in the former Soviet Union. But preparations that contain whole microbes often cause side effects, and they raise the specter that renegade cells might at times give rise to the very diseases they were meant to prevent.

The only anthrax vaccine approved for human use in the U.S. takes a different form. It consists primarily of toxin molecules that have been chemically treated to prevent them from making people ill. It is produced by growing the weakened strain of *B. anthracis* in culture, filtering the bacterial cells from the culture medium, adsorbing the toxin proteins in the remaining filtrate onto an adjuvant (a substance that enhances immune responses) and treating the mixture with formaldehyde to inactivate the proteins. Injection of this preparation, known as AVA (for anthrax vaccine adsorbed), stimulates the immune system to produce antibodies that specifically bind to and inactivate the toxin's components. Most of the antibodies act on protective antigen, however, which explains the protein's name: it is the component that best elicits protective immunity.

AVA is given to soldiers and certain civilians but is problematic as a tool for shielding the general public against biological warfare. Supplies are limited. And even if AVA were available in abundance, it would be cumbersome to deliver on a large scale; the standard protocol calls for six shots delivered over 18 months followed by annual boosters. The vaccine has not been licensed for use in people already exposed to anthrax spores. But late last year officials, worried that spores

BRYAN CHRISTIE DESIGN (*preceding two pages*)

Medical Lessons

Doctors now have a changed view of inhalation anthrax

By Ricki L. Rusting

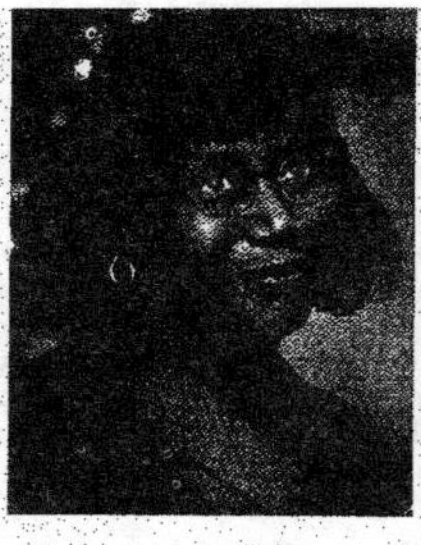

NORMA WALLACE of Willingboro, N.J., is one of the six patients who survived inhalation anthrax last autumn.

THE RECENT CASES of inhalation anthrax in the U.S. have upended some old assumptions about that disease. When contaminated letters started appearing in September 2001, public health authorities initially believed that only those who received the letters, and perhaps individuals nearby, were in danger. But spores clearly seeped out through the weave of the envelopes, contaminating postal facilities and jumping to other mail. Such "cross contamination" is a leading explanation for the deaths of two of the 11 people confirmed to have contracted inhalation anthrax last year. Also contrary to expectations, spores do not remain sedentary once they land. They can become airborne again as people walk around in a tainted room.

One surprise was positive. Before October 2001 common wisdom held that inhalation anthrax was almost always incurable after symptoms appeared. But doctors beat those odds last fall, saving six of the victims. What made the difference? Researchers cannot draw firm conclusions from so few cases. But some intriguing patterns emerged when John A. Jernigan of the Centers for Disease Control and Prevention (CDC) and a team of others reviewed the medical records of the first 10 patients. Their findings appear in the November/December 2001 *Emerging Infectious Diseases* and online at www.cdc.gov/ncidod/eid/vol7no6/jernigan.htm

Relatively prompt diagnosis may have helped, the researchers report. Inhalation anthrax has two symptomatic phases—an early period marked by maladies common to a variety of ailments (such as fatigue, fever, aches and cough) and a later phase in which patients become critically ill with high fever, labored breathing and shock. Six of the 10 patients received antibiotics active against the anthrax bacterium, *Bacillus anthracis*, while they were still showing early symptoms of infection, and only they survived.

The types of antibiotics prescribed and the use of combinations of drugs might also have had a hand in the unexpectedly high survival rate. Nine of the people discussed in the review sought care before the CDC published what it called "interim" guidelines for treating inhalation anthrax on October 26, but most patients received therapy consistent with those guidelines: ciprofloxacin (the now famous Cipro) or doxycycline plus one or two other agents known to inhibit replication of *B. anthracis* (such as rifampin, vancomycin, penicillin, ampicillin, chloramphenicol, imipenem, clindamycin and clarithromycin). Aggressive "supportive" care—including draining dangerous fluid from around the lungs—probably helped as well, scientists say.

Even the survivors were very sick, however. Jernigan says they are still being observed to see whether long-term complications will develop, although as of mid-January no obvious signs of such problems had emerged. Researchers suspect that anthrax antitoxins would ease the course of many people afflicted with anthrax and might also rescue patients who could not be saved with current therapies.

Ricki L. Rusting is a staff editor and writer.

might sometimes survive in the lungs for a long time, began offering an abbreviated, three-course dose on an experimental basis to postal workers and others who had already taken 60 days of precautionary antibiotics. People who accepted the offer were obliged to take antibiotics for an additional 40 days, after which the immunity stimulated by the vaccine would presumably be strong enough to provide adequate protection on its own.

In hopes of producing a more powerful, less cumbersome and faster-acting vaccine, many investigators are focusing on developing inoculants composed primarily of protective antigen produced by recombinant DNA technology. By coupling the recombinant protein with a potent new-generation adjuvant, scientists may be able to evoke good protective immunity relatively quickly with only one or two injections. The dominant negative inhibitors discussed earlier as possible treatments could be useful forms of protective antigen to choose. Those molecules retain their ability to elicit immune responses. Hence, they could do double duty: disarming the anthrax toxin in the short run while building up immunity that will persist later on.

We have no doubt that the expanding research on the biology of *B. anthracis* and on possible therapies and vaccines will one day provide a range of effective anthrax treatments. We fervently hope that these efforts will mean that nobody will have to die from anthrax acquired either naturally or as a result of biological terrorism. SA

MORE TO EXPLORE

Anthrax as a Biological Weapon: Medical and Public Health Management. Thomas V. Inglesby et al. in *Journal of the American Medical Association*, Vol. 281, No. 18, pages 1735–1745; May 12, 1999.

Dominant-Negative Mutants of a Toxin Subunit: An Approach to Therapy of Anthrax. Bret R. Sellman, Michael Mourez and R. John Collier in *Science*, Vol. 292, pages 695–697; April 27, 2001.

Designing a Polyvalent Inhibitor of Anthrax Toxin. Michael Mourez et al. in *Nature Biotechnology*, Vol. 19, pages 958–961; October 2001.

Identification of the Cellular Receptor for Anthrax Toxin. Kenneth A. Bradley, Jeremy Mogridge, Michael Mourez, R. John Collier and John A. T. Young in *Nature*, Vol. 414, pages 225–229; November 8, 2001.

The U.S. Centers for Disease Control and Prevention maintain a Web site devoted to anthrax at www.cdc.gov/ncidod/dbmd/diseaseinfo/anthrax_g.htm

Mr. BURTON. Thank you, Dr. Collier.

Our next witness is Dr. John Young. He's a professor in cancer research at the McArdle Laboratory for Cancer Research at the University of Wisconsin, Madison, WI.

Once again, this is your birthday. So you're recognized.

Mr. YOUNG. Thank you, Chairman Burton. It's been a pleasure to be here today, a tremendous honor for me.

Let me begin by saying that I actually got into the field of anthrax just under 3 years ago. I'm actually a virologist by training. I trained with Harold Varmus, when I was a post-doc at UCSF. Most of my lab still works on a family of viruses, retroviruses that cause cancer and AIDS.

My lab got involved in the study of anthrax in part because of my longstanding friendship with John Collier, but also over curiosity about how agents that exist outside of the cell get delivered into the interior of the cell. We were curious about the anthrax toxin receptor and how it would deliver anthrax toxin to its place of action.

So a collaborative effort was initiated between Kenneth Bradley, a graduate student in my lab, and two post-doctoral fellows in John Collier's lab, Michael Moufez and Jeremy Mogridge. They set out to clone, identify the receptor for anthrax toxin, and this work was supported by the National Institutes of Allergies and Infectious Diseases.

Now if I could have the first figure—I'm going to actually just use one figure for this presentation and take advantage of John Collier's figure 1. So, as Dr. Collier told you, the first step in anthrax intoxication is the binding of protective antigen to the cell surface, and it binds, a bit of antigen binds very specifically to this protein we've identified and called anthrax toxin receptor [ATR]. This is the docking structure for PA.

As soon as we identified this protein, this, of course, suggested to us a new, direct approach to development of another anti-toxin that was based upon this receptor, because if you can produce in large amounts the part of the receptor that normally is the docking site for PA, then that could perhaps act as an effective decoy to stop PA from sticking to the cell surface.

In fact, we've shown that that does work at least in cell culture systems. We can take cells that are growing in plastic dishes, expose them to toxin in the presence or absence of the decoy, and the decoy can protect those cells. So, at least in a culture system, in the culture conditions, this works as an anti-toxin.

We also have initiated at my lab, John Collier's lab, and with groups at Millennium Pharmaceuticals and at Biogen, have initiated a collaboration to try to produce large amounts and different types of decoy molecules to see what would be the most effective, and those studies are currently underway. Some potential decoys are being tested.

We're also in the business of trying to understand exactly how it is that PA touches down on the ATR receptor. We're going to understand the exact mechanism of recognition between these two proteins. In large part, this interest is driven out of curiosity on our part, but also it will provide in the future, we're sure, new types of therapeutic opportunities to interfere with those very specific types of interactions that these two proteins must engage in. So that work also is ongoing in the lab, and we've recently obtained new information on how these two proteins get together.

Now, in addition to studying the interaction between the receptor and the toxin, we're also very curious about the normal function and properties of this receptor. It turns out that we actually don't know what the normal function of this receptor is. It's been hijacked. It's been exploited by anthrax toxin as a means for attachment to the cell surface, but we have no idea yet what the function of this protein is.

What we do know is that the gene that encodes this protein is often upregulated in human tumors. So you'll find the gene is overexpressed in blood vessels that supply human tumors. So perhaps there's a role there for the protein in some aspect of tumor blood supply development, but we simply don't know what the normal function is at this point.

What we do know is that there is not just one form of this protein ATR. There are multiple forms of the protein, so that we show one model up there, one protein that spans the membrane once, but we've identified several different, what we call, isoforms or different forms of the protein. We would like to understand what they do. Do they interact with anthrax toxin? And if they do, do they also lead to subsequent intoxication of the cell?

So understanding the protein in more detail, the different forms of the protein, understanding some of the steps that are outlined in figure 1 by arrows here, what's shown here is a sequential step of events that must occur for intoxication to take place. We would like to understand what the role of the receptor is in getting this seven-membered ring with its cargo loaded onto it to the right place in the cell for that toxin to be delivered very effectively into the cell, so it can begin its toxic actions. This is essentially what we can in scientific terms call uptake and trafficking of these complexities to the site of action.

So there is a lot of basic science in my lab aimed at trying to understand exactly how that process is controlled. Again, our goal is to understand the biology of this system in greater detail, but, undoubtedly, if we can do that, then, of course, that's going to offer new types of therapeutic approaches in the future, we believe, aimed at stopping those other aspects of the toxin entry pathway.

So I'd actually just like to sum up at this point. When thinking about quickening the pace in anthrax toxin research, I think we have to think about this from two different perspectives. I think what we have to do is we have to look at the exciting new approaches that are available now, antibodies against protective antigen, these decoy types of proteins, these types of inhibitors that Dr. Collier mentioned, the polyvalent inhibitor, dominant negative inhibitor. These are agents that are available now and can be tested in animal model systems if these animal model systems become easily available to test them in.

But I think we have to really think more broadly about how we're going to approach not just anthrax toxin, but any type of bioweapon agent that might be delivered, using similar mechanisms to those shown on this slide. I think for that we really have to rely upon the entire scientific community to better understand some of these very basic properties in the cell, these early steps that allow cargo to be taken up from the outside and delivered to the inside.

We've made some remarkable progress, again because of the insight and support of NIH. The community has made tremendous progress understanding these processes, but we need to understand them in much greater detail if we are going to figure out very smart ways that we can stop pathogenic organisms from exploiting those pathways that the cell needs for its normal functions. So I really think that we have to think very, very broadly about how we go about doing this.

With respect to that, too, it should be clear from what I said previously that with the anthrax toxin receptor, here's a gene that's upregulated in tumor blood supply. On the one hand, you wouldn't equate the two areas of scientific discipline. You wouldn't say that tumor blood supply is going to give you any insight into a treatment for anthrax toxin, but it may, in fact, be that understanding what the normal function of this receptor is will suggest some future therapies that could be used against this agent and others.

So I'll close there and thank you.

[The prepared statement of Mr. Young follows:]

Full Committee Hearing on "Quickening the Pace of Research in Protecting Against Anthrax and Other Biological Terrorist Agents-A Look at Toxin Interference"

John A.T. Young, Ph.D.
Written Testimony
February 22, 2002

My laboratory, in a collaboration with Dr. John Collier's group at Harvard Medical School, recently identified ATR, the long-elusive cellular receptor for anthrax toxin. ATR binds directly to the protective antigen (PA) component of anthrax toxin to facilitate the first step of intoxication. We have identified the region of the receptor that binds to PA. Furthermore, we have produced a free-floating region of the receptor, designated as soluble ATR (sATR), which is an effective decoy that prevents PA from binding to cell surfaces. Thus, sATR is an attractive candidate anti-toxin which may be useful for the treatment of anthrax. Moreover, the cloning of the receptor now makes it possible to screen for drugs that specifically block the interaction between PA and ATR.

Current research within my laboratory, and in collaboration with Dr. Collier's group and with Dr. Mogridge's group at the University of Toronto, is aimed at characterizing: 1. The specific molecular interactions between PA and ATR; 2. How the PA-receptor interactions lead to toxin uptake into cells; 3. The site within the cell where the active components of the toxin (edema factor and lethal factor) are delivered so that they can perform their toxic functions. These studies will provide new insights into the cell biology of anthrax toxin uptake into cells and could provide future novel therapeutic opportunities tc treat the disease.

We are also attempting to understand what is the normal function of ATR. Although this is not yet known, expression of the ATR gene is specifically up-regulated in the blood vessels that help support the growth of human tumors. Thus, by studying this receptor we may also gain a deeper understanding of processes involved in the establishment and progression of cancer. Most importantly, by knowing the natural function of the receptor, we should be able to design receptor-based therapeutic strategies that specifically inhibit toxin action, thereby reducing the possibility of any toxic side-effects of treatment.

High levels of toxin, that accompany the onset of symptoms after inhalation exposure to anthrax bacterial spores, most likely contribute to death even if antibiotics are administered to prevent new rounds of bacterial growth. Therefore, it is imperative that antitoxin approaches be tested as soon as possible in animal model systems for their efficacy in preventing death due to anthrax. It is possible that a combination therapy consisting of antibiotics and a "cocktail" of anti-toxins will prove useful in preventing death even at a stage when symptoms have developed. Such a combination therapy may also prove useful against a variety of different *Bacillus anthracis* strains, even those that have been engineered to be antibiotic-resistant or vaccine-resistant.

Mr. BURTON. Thank you very much, Dr. Young. Are you from Ireland, Scotland, or Australia?

Mr. YOUNG. Actually, I'm from Scotland, but I have been in this country for almost 15 years now.

Mr. BURTON. I thought Scotland. My son and I were over there playing golf not long ago, and you sounded like one of those people that we talked to over there, very nice people. [Laughter.]

I don't like haggis though.

Let me start off the questioning by asking, first of all, and Dr. Smith and I had a chance to talk before we had the hearing today, and I think you indicated, Dr. Smith, that at some point you think it's possible that people who are exposed to inhalation anthrax might be able to use some kind of a spray that would immediately inhibit that from becoming toxic to the human body.

I think the first question for all of you, and I'll start with you, Dr. Smith, is: How long will it take, roughly, if the funds are adequate for research, how long will it take before we have some kind of a solution to this problem that the American people, the mass of American people, could count on? I mean, we're talking about the possibility of a massive attack in an urban area down the road from these terrorist groups that are around the world. So can you give us a timeframe and what type of spray or vaccination could we come up with that would be effective, not only against anthrax but against Ebola and other types of toxic substances?

Mr. SMITH. Thank you, Mr. Chairman. Through the History Channel, I'd like to make a comparison. I didn't realize that the Pentagon as a building was built in 1 year, but that was during a time at the very beginning of World War II. It will take far more time than that to get it back in shape after one plane hitting it.

It's the speed at which we want to see something done; it is directed by the speed which we put behind it. I think from the protease inhibitor approach, as I said in my presentation, the Chloromethylketone, which is in the literature as a means of stopping infection, that has been done, but that compound cannot be used as a drug candidate. It would take from 90 to 120 days, by the judgment of the synthesis chemists in enzyme systems products, to synthesize a first-generation inhibitor that could be handed, for example, to Dr. Thomas to run through tissue culture work and the elegant work that he has done in the past, to evaluate that to see if it then could be carried on to the other very competent gentlemen here to run in animal models.

The whole thing could be done, in my opinion, in less than a year's time, if there was the funding behind it. It's no more funding to do that than to delay it, because the amount of funding to make these compounds is not great.

I had the privilege to talk to Beth yesterday and said that it actually would be the cost of about one penny to every American citizen to fund that type of research. I think that answers itself.

Mr. BURTON. And we'll go down the panel with that question. So you think that within a year, if the resources were available and everybody got to work on this, that we could come up with not only some kind of approach for dealing with the anthrax threat, but also with these other threats as well?

Mr. SMITH. Possibly with—now anthrax could be used, anthrax inhibitor is seen of a molecule that is less than a thousand molecular weight. That means it's extremely small. It would be about the size of a golf ball compared to the anthrax bacteria itself, which would be more like the size of a basketball. So your drug in this particular case is much smaller than the organism.

The antibody approach, or even the elegant mutated or designed natural molecules, are about a hundred times larger, in the 30,000 to 40,000 molecular weight range. I believe, preempting Dr. Balhorn, that he has some work that will ultimately show the difference and what that could mean in how fast we approach something.

Mr. BURTON. Dr. Thomas.

Mr. THOMAS. Well, thank you. It certainly would seem to me to develop novel strategies for anthrax that would be optical to people certainly would take some time. I would think that part of this would depend certainly on funding, but another is bringing together a team of talented scientists with different expertise from peptide or small molecule design, for example, to sub-biology-type assays, to animal studies, that I think can run through a number of assays that I think are probably fairly well established in labs around the country—at NIH, for example—to begin testing these.

How long that takes is always tough, I think, to answer because you do go into animal models and you do go into unknowns. It's the mystery of science as to how long this can go on for, but I would imagine, certainly from the panel's discussion that I've listened to this afternoon, this is something that I think is compelling, and I think it's imminent, that in fact progress can be made to alternative strategies probably within just a short few years' time. Certainly the collaboration between scientists and corporations I think is of great benefit to some of these approaches, and so I think that certainly parts of this are well on the way to seeing some success. That's for anthrax.

Then for the broader development, for example, other targets, whether we use a protease inhibitor of the kind that I described or new-generation protease inhibitors, I think really depends upon the team and the talent that we can recruit into this area. Certainly the talent is available around the country to do this. It's a matter of assembling that talent in an organized way in a mission such that we do attain that goal, and I think in just a few short years.

Mr. BURTON. Let me interrupt and just say this.

Mr. YOUNG. Yes, sir.

Mr. BURTON. I'm sure that NIH knows how to get this done.

Mr. YOUNG. Yes.

Mr. BURTON. Those of us on this panel are neophytes as far as this kind of information goes and how to deal with it, but what I would like for you to do as panelists, and you don't have to do this today, but I'd like for you to give me your best advice on the length of time that you think this would take, No. 1, a rough idea, and I'm sure it's going to vary; the amount of money that you think it might cost, and I know again that's probably going to be something you're going to have to pull out of the air, but you've dealt with this before so you have some idea of what research costs, and then what kind of a team we'd have to put together. If I could get that information from you and the other panelists who are going to be here today—do we have anybody here from NIH today? Would you raise your hand?

I'm sure that we could convey that to them, and I'm sure they're very receptive to that kind of information, and we could get on with this as quickly as possible. I'm not sure, and I don't think anybody knows, how long we have before the next terrorist attack, if one does occur. But the one thing that I'm pretty confident of, if we have one, it's going to be probably as bad or worse than what we saw before. If it's a bioterrorist attack, it could end up killing tens of thousands or hundreds of thousands or more. So time is of the essence.

So if you have information or judgments that you could give to us that we could convey to our friends at NIH who are here today, maybe we could cut through some of this paperwork and some of this bureaucracy that we deal with here in the Congress, to get to the heart of the matter as quickly as possible. No. 1, get you the money you need. No. 2, help you to assemble the technicians and the scientists that are necessary to come up with a solution, maybe cut through the time that's required for the lab tests with the animals, and so forth, so that we could get this thing prepared and ready for the population on a massive scale before we have that kind of terrorist attack.

So I just hope that you'll give this committee that information, and at the same time it will be going to NIH, and then we can kind of maybe work together to make sure we get the funding and everything else that's necessary.

Dr. Collier.

Mr. COLLIER. I have very little to add to what Dr. Thomas and Dr. Smith said. It's very difficult to estimate with any accuracy how long it will take to develop any given drug. We have a number of candidates already on the table. There are companies and laboratories now screening libraries of compounds for inhibitory activity to block toxin agent.

From what I showed on the slide, you can see that there are many, many steps in the action of this toxin. Potentially any one of those can be interfered with. We can go after the inhibitors either by a rational approach or by screening enormous numbers of compounds that might inhibit one or another step, and both of those need to be done and are being done.

I think Dr. Smith didn't—the focus has been on the furin, inhibiting furin as a step in proteolytic activation of PA. I don't think he has mentioned also that the lethal factor is also a protease, metalla-protease. So this is another step or another target of the action of seeking inhibitors.

I know at least one major drug company that's now doing very high throughput screening of their large battery of compounds for ability to inhibit the lethal factor action. I think I'll stop there and turn the floor over to Dr. Young.

Mr. BURTON. Dr. Young.

Mr. YOUNG. I actually have nothing really more to add in terms of timeframe. I think it's almost impossible to estimate with any reasonably certainty when there will be an effective anti-toxin on the table.

I think that one thing that's quite clear, though, in the last 5 months, having gone to various institutions across the country and given seminars, that many scientists who, like me, were not involved in this area of research want to get involved. They really want to get involved. They want to do something. In order for them to do something, they have to have resources. I have no idea how to put a dollar figure on what kind of activity that would take, but it's quite clear that very creative people, chemists, biologists, from many different types of disciplines with very different skills—we think about problems in different types of ways—want to make a difference here.

So my only suggestion then would be to make sure that they could do so without any barrier whatsoever, financial or a resource. I think that if there's a barrier in place, it's going to hold people back from really jumping in and trying something that's new, which I think might, in fact, be the difference.

Anti-toxins that are on the table today may not look like the anti-toxins of the future. I think the sooner we get to that stage of having the most effective drugs and products on the table, the better position we'll be in to deal with any bioterrorist threat. So that's the only thing I would say about that.

Mr. BURTON. Let me say, before I yield to my colleagues, whatever it takes, we'll be glad to help you with to cut through the red tape necessary to get answers as quickly as possible, because I don't think anybody in the Congress doubts that we have to do this as expeditiously as we possibly can, get it done. We just don't want to see Indianapolis or Chicago or Los Angeles or New York suffer 100,000 casualties because we didn't get on this as quickly as possible.

Connie, do you have a comment?

Mrs. MORELLA. Thanks, Mr. Chairman. Since Mr. Shays yielded to me, he had no question, and Mr. Weldon will be back in the room.

Thank you for calling this hearing. I'm glad I'm not being given a test on explaining exactly your material. [Laughter.]

But in terms of the general policy provisions, this is what we are here for. Last year the FDA approved the antibiotic Cipro, a previously licensed product for the new indication of treating inhalation anthrax based on animal studies. Cipro had been tested in humans for other indications, and it was shown to be safe and effective.

Developing new drugs that will protect against anthrax and other biological terrorism agents really presents some specific testing challenges, and that's what I will be asking because, how will we develop these drugs and test them adequately, since it's not ethical to intentionally expose human beings to inhalation anthrax to see if the treatment works? Do you think, therefore, following up on that, as you respond, do you think that there should be a different level of evidence that would be needed to approve these products, such as that proposed animal rule which would allow the FDA to approve a new drug that is effective against inhalation anthrax based only on animal data? I address it to anybody, anybody who wants to——

Mr. SMITH. May I be the first to respond then? In the case of the small molecular weight inhibitors, which obviously I champion—I champion them on the basis that, as I said, they have proven successful in the treatment of HIV infection, and there are in pre-clinical trials of these inhibitors at some of the major universities for the enzymes called caspase in the treatment of the disease states that I talked to, such as Parkinson's disease, ALS, Huntington's, and stroke, the furin inhibitors aren't too far removed from them. They're small molecules, and they require—just simply the first line of testing is to test in cell cultures the elegant systems which Dr. Thomas' laboratory has established.

Dr. Thomas and I have discussed this in some detail by ourselves and in the presence of Beth Clay as well, as to how we would pursue this by doing this where no animals are involved, no humans are involved. If it doesn't pass muster there, then the technology is no good. If it does, you move on sequentially.

Of course, the more positives you have, the faster you can build-up your data base, because of your condition to move quicker. I still think that the very original development of the chemistry—wet chemistry, as we refer to it—can be done within a year period of time. I'm not agating the amount of time that it would take would be longer to go through the cellular work and into the animal work; that's a given, and there are certain requirements and specific things that have to be met in accordance to the Food and Drug Administration and the NIH to do those type of investigations, but I think it's plausible.

Mrs. MORELLA. Would any of the rest of our distinguished panelists, like to comment on that? I think that was a recommendation, an animal rule recommendation, that I think had not been followed through. Maybe this is something I should be asking the next panel, but I would like to get your comments on the testing problem.

Mr. THOMAS. I think this is where I also become a layperson in some of these areas, but what the committee is doing is really pushing scientists very hard for taking cutting-edge science in biological research that I think you've heard here today and translating that into new drug therapies. That's why I think you're picking up some caution on the committee, because we are talking about research, basic science research, that, in fact, we are compelled, like you, to see how we could translate some of our basic new findings of how cells function, how pathogens function, into new drugs.

It's slightly different, for example, than coming up with a new sleeping pill at a major pharmaceutical company, where you have ideas on how to escape patent issues with competition somewhere else, but this is something different. This is where, in fact, it does always hold additional research that we need to do as we come into these areas. This is why I think you're picking up caution, and appropriately so, from the committee members, that in fact you do have to take this in steps and go through cell work, go through animal work.

This is why it's tough to give you an exact time on when something is due, because what you're asking for is some translation of just new findings in cell function and how that can translate into a therapy and how fast we could do that. Those are tough because we really are pushing the envelope of what we're finding for new discoveries on how those functions.

Mrs. MORELLA. Since I think I have a little more time left, then I'm going to avail myself of asking maybe our other two panelists, what specific recommendations would you make to the DOD and NIH today? Being on the first panel, you don't have a chance to interact with the second panel. So this might be your opportunity to offer whatever you would like.

Mr. COLLIER. I guess I would simply reiterate two of the points that I made in my initial presentation: that, No. 1, there's a major need to find new models or models that will really work in accelerating the development through government/corporate partnerships rapidly. As I said, it appears to me that DARPA has a viable model for doing that, with allowing an appropriate amount of money to be directed to a project, overseeing the project with a manager that will have flexibility and ability to keep close tabs on the project, be sure it's moving very rapidly.

I'm a layperson as well in trying to think about these things, but I have not seen other models in the government institutions that we've spoken with that are perhaps as close to this as one might like. So that would be, I think, the major point that I would make.

Mrs. MORELLA. OK. Dr. Young, do you want to add anything?

Mr. COLLIER. Pardon?

Mrs. MORELLA. No, thank you, Dr. Collier.

Mr. COLLIER. Yes, sorry.

Mrs. MORELLA. I was going to then recognize Dr. Young.

Mr. YOUNG. Well, if Dr. Collier feels like a layperson in this area, I feel like a level below that in this area. I think that——

Mrs. MORELLA. You're making me all feel pretty good. [Laughter.]

Mr. YOUNG. It's quite clear, though, that even with existing antitoxins on the table, that there are some major roadblocks, and have been major roadblocks, to having those products produced in large amounts and tested in appropriate model systems.

I think that one of the big lessons for me in the last 6 months or so has been learning not how much we know about anthrax and the pathogenesis of the disease, but how little we know about this. Despite remarkable progress that's been made by a number of investigators in this field, we actually know remarkably little about biology of the spore, for example. We know remarkably little about how it is that people end up dying from this disease.

I think that when thinking about model systems, animal model systems, and advising the DOD or NIH about model systems, which model system is going to most closely mimic that of a human? You have to find something that is most closely related to the human condition, but we don't know much about what it is that we're looking for in that model system, because we don't understand the disease in humans well enough to really know that.

So I think that really, again, my advice in this area is to think broadly. A number of systems may have to be tried, tested. They might not work. Test them as quickly as you possibly can, get the information, and move on. Don't sit on your hands, scientists sit on their hands, not the people on the panel there—scientists don't sit on their hands. Get things done; get information, and then get our heads together and figure out exactly how it is that we can create the best model system for this disease. Then ensure that people who have novel and creative approaches are allowed to develop them and have them tested in short order to see if they can then be translated into a product that can be used in humans.

Mrs. MORELLA. Thank you. I want to thank the panel.

Dr. Young, have you ever met Dr. Frank Young, who previously was an FDA Director? I know my NIH people are kind of smiling affirmatively. Have you ever met him?

Mr. YOUNG. No.

Mrs. MORELLA. No?

He had testified before a Science Committee I'm on on bioterrorism and the testing situation. With the same name, I just thought that you might have, and in similar fields. Thank you.

Thank you, Mr. Chairman.

Mr. BURTON. Thank you, Mrs. Morella. Mr. Shays. Mr. Horn.

Mr. HORN. Thank you very much, Mr. Chairman. I came in from other activities, and I didn't hear the first part, but I notice this little box here of the anthrax protective antigen. I thought that since my colleagues have it, that maybe we'll have a seniority change on this panel. [Laughter.]

What will activate, if anything, the anthrax protective antigen, can you inject it in some human or is it a spray that you can do it? Give me some layman's response on that.

Mr. SMITH. Well, if that's in reference to anthrax that would be inhaled, that there is a possibility with low-molecular weight inhibitors that they could, subsequently, within a matter of the most convenient and most expeditious time period, with an inhaling mechanism inhaled the potential protective antigen inhibitor because it is such a small molecule. In other disease states, where the furin enzyme plays a very important role, I think it would probably have to ultimately be injected in some form, especially if you were trying to ward off an Ebola attack.

Mr. HORN. Any other comments on this? Dr. Collier.

Mr. COLLIER. Yes. With regard to the inhibitors described, these are large molecules. Our thinking is that they probably would have to be injected. Possibly a spray delivery system might be developed or possibly even enteric pill that you could swallow, but at this point our thinking is that it's likely that they would have to be injected, yes.

Mr. HORN. Dr. Young, do you have any thoughts on this?

Mr. YOUNG. I have nothing to add other than what Dr. Collier has already said.

Mr. HORN. Does the drug development research have to be conducted in a B–4 level laboratory? That's the highest level, is it not, in handling this, or this very difficult to spread it out? How many laboratories do you think could do this and work with this? We know Harvard can. We know Wisconsin can. We know NIH can. What is going on in Europe on this? What do we know as scientists? Are you all waiting for the Nobel Prize? [Laughter.]

You're not playing any cards.

Mr. COLLIER. Probably Dr. Friedlander on the next panel might be best equipped to answer this, but there are only two or three places, Art, in the country that can handle inhalational anthrax that are equipped to do those types of experiments. What we badly need is possibly a single center in the country with much greater capacity. Capacity to do the appropriate experiments needed to test these compounds, there's a major roadblock there that needs to be overcome. I know that NIH is thinking about this; CDC is thinking about this, and I'm sure the Army. But this is something that really needs to be considered.

Mr. HORN. Now is this a vaccine that we're headed for more than that? Let's say you have—I'm going to Nashville tomorrow, and we're going to have data on chemical attacks, biological attacks, nuclear, etc. We're doing that in a number of cities across America, just to alert people that what are the things one can do. So I would be curious what would be things that people can do, the local sheriff, the local public health authorities, the hospitals in the area. What would you suggest the kind of questions we ought to pry to see if something happens and the people in Nashville, say, have something in the water system?

Mr. COLLIER. Well, I think you should tell them that we're working avidly on all of these approaches. The panel today is concentrating mostly on therapeutic approach to anthrax. We have heard a number of candidates put forward, and a number of others are being thought about.

Vaccine, new types of vaccines are being developed and being considered. In fact, the NIH has an initiative now to do a very fast-track development of a new vaccine. Beyond that, I don't know how to recommend what you should say to the folks in Nashville.

Mr. HORN. Nashville, Milwaukee, we're looking at the medium-sized cities. The big cities, New York and Dallas and all of the 1 million or more, they usually have fairly good emergency management and public health, but we want to see what else is happening. Because when you add all the others up, you're talking about millions of people.

Dr. Young.

Mr. YOUNG. Yes, I think the message should really be that the existing vaccine, while effective, obviously, has complications. There are new types of vaccines already in the pipeline, at least one that's being pushed hard at the moment to be tested.

But, undoubtedly, as more and more people get involved in this type of research, then the whole area of vaccine development will also be one that will go through some form of evolution. It will change from perhaps its current state into a new one that might be more effective.

So I think the message to the people of Nashville should be that scientists are working very hard on trying to come up with ways to develop an effective vaccine with minimum side effects.

Mr. HORN. Dr. Smith, how long does it take to develop the products necessary to test for toxin interference?

Mr. SMITH. The small molecular type inhibitors are done, as I've tried to articulate, by what is laboratory simple chemistry, where you use flasks and beakers and reagents of that nature in an organic synthesis type of setting. There are many major pharmaceutical companies that do this. There are several pharmaceutical companies that presently are making HIV protease inhibitors and marketing them, as I'm sure you know. This is a continuation of that concept, and if we can take that same approach, only not attacking the organism, the HIV or the anthrax, but attacking the part of the cell—and if it won't split the protective antigen, it cannot infect. We try to avoid that split. If we can do that, we have made it. If we can't, we have failed. It's a simple yes-or-no answer.

Mr. HORN. Dr. Leppla's written testimony states that there are at least eight distinct phases in which the anthrax toxin may be interrupted. Why have you selected the furin interference as the stage to develop?

Mr. SMITH. Because it's the first cellular organelle entry, etc., that the anthrax organism sees. To be sure, as Dr. Collier said, there is another enzyme within the cell which is known as the lethal factor. It is a protease as well, but it involves a different type of protease called a metalla-protease, and those proteases are down the line. It's not the first line of defense. It would have to be defined as the second line of defense.

Mr. HORN. Do you think the other stages should be explored simultaneously?

Mr. SMITH. Well, certainly. I wouldn't leave out vaccines although I'm not a devotee of vaccines.

Mr. HORN. What about other medical conditions that are likely to benefit from the research conducted on the anthrax anti-toxin?

Mr. SMITH. I think Dr. Thomas stated it very eloquently: the various forms of cancer, the various other types of infectious disease from measles to cytomegalovirus to mononucleosis. There are different types of kissing cousins, so to speak: the Marbur virus to the Ebola viruses. All of these could in one form or another cause minimal concern by causing havoc by just diphtheria or measles epidemic.

Mr. HORN. What other biological agents act similarly to anthrax that we might develop treatments in a similar fashion?

Mr. SMITH. Well, the interesting thing about these inhibitors is that they are extremely specific. By changing just single amino acids within a protein to accommodate a particular organism, one gets a degree of specificity, and we don't know today how extensive that specificity can be.

Mr. HORN. Now we've got currently an outbreak of Ebola in the Congo. Could we possibly develop a treatment that would be effective both for protection against a terrorist threat and to help outbreaks of Ebola in the Congo and the other African nations?

Mr. SMITH. With the appropriate synthetic protease inhibitor, I think there is a good possibility. I certainly couldn't give you a guarantee, but I think it's route of treatment would not be inhalation or topical as would be in the case of anthrax, but would have to be intravenous injection since the Ebola virus works in a very different way in its killing process, by destroying the liver and blood vessels.

Mr. BURTON. Mr. Horn, can we catch you on the next round?

Mr. HORN. All right, this last question is——

Mr. BURTON. OK, sir.

Mr. HORN [continuing]. Are we working on this in the United States or in Europe?

Mr. SMITH. We've done some limited work and have theorized on paper what these inhibitors should look like chemistry-wise, but I don't know of anyone personally anywhere else in the whole world who has done it yet, besides ourselves.

Mr. HORN. Well, I thank you for your judgments on this. It's very important.

Mr. BURTON. Thank you, Mr. Horn.

Mr. Thomas, you indicated while Dr. Smith was talking that you might have something that you wanted to add real quickly. Did you have something you'd like to——

Mr. THOMAS. It was just a followup, but I think Dr. Smith handled it very well: that why to go after furin is it really represents, I think, the tip of an iceberg for the activation of a number of bacterial and viral pathogens, as well as a number of human diseases. We went through a couple of examples, including rheumatoid arthritis and metastatic cancer. It's, in fact, those reasons why I think that targeting furin could have potentially broad application for a broad-based therapeutic. But I think it was answered eloquently enough by Dr. Smith.

Mr. BURTON. Thank you.

Dr. Weldon.

Dr. WELDON. I want to thank the chairman. My occupation before coming here was I practiced medicine. I still see patients once a month, internal medicine, and I actually did infectious disease for about 7 years. My undergraduate degree is in biochemistry.

This is fascinating, Mr. Chairman, bringing these people in here and to hear this kind of research. It's fascinating to see how sophisticated our knowledge and understanding has emerged at least over the last 20 years since I was a college student.

Let me just understand correctly this model, Dr. Collier. You arranged to have this provided to us, correct? Is that right? And it was made by Dr. Herman in Milwaukee, is that correct?

Mr. COLLIER. Yes, yes.

Dr. WELDON. This is a model of the protective antigen with—and it's normally heptamer-7——

Mr. COLLIER. Yes.

Dr. WELDON [continuing]. Protective antigens that are linked together and then put in this one; the white one is the one that has some amino acids altered.

Mr. COLLIER. Yes.

Dr. WELDON. And this is one of the concepts that you have for a drug treatment, correct?

Mr. COLLIER. That's correct.

Dr. WELDON. Why is it called protective antigen? That is very confusing. I don't know who picked that name, but I would highly suggest you change the name. [Laughter.]

Because it's protecting edema factor and lethal factor, is that why they gave it that kind of a name?

Mr. COLLIER. No, this is a name that emerged way back in the 1950's, I guess.

Dr. WELDON. In the 1950's?

Mr. COLLIER. Yes, when the protein was first discovered. It's the part of the toxin that induces protective antibodies in the body, the most effective one.

Dr. WELDON. So that's how it was given that name?

Mr. COLLIER. That's how it got its name, yes. We might name it a little bit differently now——

Dr. WELDON. This is nasty stuff, correct? I mean, this is——

Mr. COLLIER. In actual fact, the protein itself by itself, as far as one can tell, is not toxic at all, unless it has the other two.

Dr. WELDON. It needs the other two?

Mr. COLLIER. Yes.

Dr. WELDON. Now the patient comes in, is diagnosed with inhaled anthrax, is given antibiotics, but ends up dying anyway because in some cases the bacterial load in the bloodstream is so high that they're going to die of shock, no matter what. But in some of them it's because the body burden of lethal factor and edema factor and this injection mechanism is so high that, even though you've killed and eradicated all the active bacteria in their body with antibiotics, with high-dose antibiotics, this stuff is going to kill them anyway, correct?

Mr. COLLIER. That's the current thinking.

Dr. WELDON. OK. And your thinking is, by introducing, either through injection or through a tablet form you mentioned, something like the white one here, it would just interfere with the whole pathophysiologic mechanism that's involved in the terminal phase of the disease?

Mr. COLLIER. That's the hope, and at what stage, obviously, at some point in the stage the patient can't be rescued; no question. So how late in the course of the disease something like this inhibitor could be administered and still save the patient is right now anybody's guess.

Dr. WELDON. OK. And, Dr. Young, you said, I think, in your presentation the other idea, other than having a genetically engineered variant of the protective antigen, is to approach it several other ways to block the mechanism of injection with smaller molecules, correct? And you've mentioned the peptide, I think?

Mr. YOUNG. Yes. Actually, it could be done with either antibodies that we bind to protective antigen and stop it from binding to cell surfaces or it can be done with a decoy type of protein I described.

Dr. WELDON. Right.

Mr. YOUNG. Small molecules that would disrupt that interaction have not been discovered yet, but, obviously, that would be a goal for future research, to find something like that.

I think that an important thing to bring up is that the lesson from HIV has been you must use a cocktail of inhibitors if you want to really, as effectively as you can, stop——

Dr. WELDON. Shut it off?

Mr. YOUNG [continuing]. Shut off the process. So it may be, in fact, that one anti-toxin isn't going to be sufficient. You may have to target the eight steps that Dr. Leppla has outlined, eight different steps of this process, to get really effective blockage of toxin action.

Dr. WELDON. Right.

Mr. YOUNG. But the strategies that target the steps on the outside of the cell are just much more accessible——

Dr. WELDON. Sure.

Mr. YOUNG [continuing]. Than those inside the cell. So that's why they're attractive as a first step in this process.

Dr. WELDON. Now, Dr. Thomas, if I understand you correctly, the furin enzyme is necessary for the formation of these proteins, is that correct?

Mr. THOMAS. Yes, so the furin pathway, the furin enzyme is necessary for activating the larger form of protective antigen. When the bacterium releases protective antigen, it releases it as a larger inactive protein, and it has to be cut by furin to generate the smaller active form that can form as heptamer. So the idea would be for furin inhibitors is, if you block furin, then you block the ability of this protective antigen to form this heptamer that can produce a syringe-like quality.

Dr. WELDON. So the anthrax has released all of this protein in the bloodstream that has protective antigen in it, and the furin on the cell surface is actually cleaving that protein to produce the active form of this? So your theory is, if you can block the cell surface furin, that's another potential way to block the toxic cascade essentially?

Mr. THOMAS. Exactly.

Dr. WELDON. OK. Are you getting enough research funding, all of you? We talked a little bit about this. Most of you, I would assume, are funded by NIH or one of its affiliated agencies. With more funding, you could accelerate your work? Is that what you're telling us here today? I know every scientist says that, but——

Mr. THOMAS. I think it would be——

Dr. WELDON. Pardon me?

Mr. THOMAS. I'm sorry, I didn't mean to interrupt. I was just going to mention I think it would be rare to find a scientist who says he's adequately funded nowadays.

Dr. WELDON. Right.

Mr. THOMAS. But in the context of our work, we are funded by NIDDK. We were funded originally by NIDDK, that led to the funding or led to the invention of the furin inhibitor that I did describe this morning. That actually translated into research that was subsequently funded by NIAID on basic questions on cytomegalovirus assembly.

But, specifically, on the PDX inhibitor that I've described for you and the various uses of it, in fact, we're not funded on it currently, but it's something that we're preparing for in the laboratory, for doing.

Dr. WELDON. So you plan to apply for grants to help something like this?

Mr. THOMAS. Sure, certainly.

Dr. WELDON. Did you say that you've done some toxicology studies on the PDX inhibitor that——

Mr. THOMAS. Yes, there has been some short-term toxicity studies done in rats by a couple of groups, taking the PDX, and through injection, and they found no short-term acute toxicity with this reagent.

The reagent right now is made in bacteria. So it has a fairly short half-life in the animal. So we think that to increase its bioavailability would mean that we would change the ways in which we would make PDX. We would make new generations of this inhibitor.

But one potential use of this, particularly thinking in terms of anthrax, is that we did build this inhibitor based on a scaffold of a protein that's well characterized called Alpha–1 Antitrypsin, certainly with its roles in emphysema, for example. A lot of the pharmacokinetics of Alpha–1 Antitrypsin are fairly well-established, and it's known, coincidentally, to concentrate in the lung.

Dr. WELDON. Right.

Mr. THOMAS. So maybe there's a possibility that, by a second-generation-type inhibitor that we're developing, that we could maybe have one that's more bioavailable, longer-lasting that would target the lung, and maybe we would see some success in this area. But this is something that just hasn't been done yet. So we don't know.

Dr. WELDON. Now if I understand you correctly, and I think the next witnesses are going to elaborate on this more, vaccination of the whole population would be very difficult. We could probably vaccinate first-responders, but if we were not to vaccinate the whole population, we would need other drugs to help us in the setting of a mass outbreak because, clearly, antibiotics given late don't always work; you can still lose people. That's where these products could find an application.

If I understand you correctly, you feel very strongly that they could have applications in the management of cancer as well, correct?

Mr. THOMAS. Yes, we think so. We see certainly some preliminary data and some very simple animal models that, in fact, we can block metastasis by blocking this particular pathway. The cascade that furin initiates that leads to tumor metastasis I think is fairly well understood because it activates actually multiple protease systems that themselves have been allowed tumors to metastasize and invade other tissues.

In fact, with colleagues at the Fox-Chase Cancer Center, they have been able to show that, if they use this particular reagent that we've developed, that in a very simple animal model, mind you, they still can block the metastatic potential of these tumor cells. So it's a proof of concept, in fact, that——

Dr. WELDON. Yes, I found it very interesting, actually, when you presented that to us. Have you presented that information at any of the cancer meetings?

Mr. THOMAS. I think that my colleague, Dr. Andres Klein-Szanto at the Fox-Chase Cancer Center has presented this at several meetings this last year, and it was recently published in the National Academy of Sciences this past fall.

Dr. WELDON. Great. Thank you very much, Mr. Chairman.

Mr. BURTON. Unless there's further questions, we'll thank this panel very much for your expertise and your testimony. Before you leave, let me just, once again, ask you to, if you have some suggestions on funding or research or team research, or things that we've talked about here today, I wish you would not only convey those to NIH, but also to Beth on our committee, so that we can do what we can to help do whatever it is possible to get additional funding for the research that's necessary.

In particular, this area of metastatic cancer you're talking about, I have a personal experience with my family with that right now. I want to tell you, there's so many people in this country that have been just devastated by the metastasizing of cancer, that it's not funny. Boy, I'll tell you, I wish you all the success in the world in getting that research done as quickly as possible, in addition to the research on these other things.

So thank you very much. I want to thank all the panel.

We'll now bring our next panel forward. Our next panel consists of: Dr. Rodney Balhorn, he's research director at Lawrence Livermore Laboratories; Dr. Stephen Leppla, he's the senior investigator for the National Institute of Dental and Cranial Facial Research of the National Institute of Health in Bethesda; Dr. Arthur Friedlander, he's a senior scientist in the U.S. Army Medical Research Institute of Infectious Diseases at Fort Detrick, MD.

Would you please stand, so we can swear you in? This is a common practice we do here. I don't think it needs to be done today, but we'll follow that common practice.

[Witnesses sworn.]

Mr. BURTON. Be seated.

I think we'll go right down the list here. Dr. Balhorn, would you like to make an opening statement, sir?

STATEMENTS OF RODNEY BALHORN, RESEARCH DIRECTOR, LAWRENCE LIVERMORE LABORATORIES, DEPARTMENT OF ENERGY, LIVERMORE, CA; STEPHEN LEPPLA, SENIOR INVESTIGATOR FOR THE NATIONAL INSTITUTE OF DENTAL AND CRANIAL FACIAL RESEARCH, NATIONAL INSTITUTE OF HEALTH, BETHESDA, MD; AND ARTHUR FRIEDLANDER, SENIOR SCIENTIST, U.S. ARMY MEDICAL RESEARCH INSTITUTE OF INFECTIOUS DISEASES, FORT DETRICK, FREDERICK, MD

Mr. BALHORN. Yes, I would. Thank you very much for the invitation, and for giving me a chance to speak.

I think the panel that spoke before us, at least from my point of view, set the stage very well for what I would like to describe. They told you a lot about several different approaches that can be used to design new inhibitors to block anthrax toxin, and minimize its effectiveness.

What we have been doing at Lawrence Livermore National Lab, in collaboration with other National Labs, as part of the Chemical and Biological National Security Program, is to design very specialized, small molecules that target and attach to specific sites on proteins, and this approach could be applied directly to inhibitor design. What we are currently doing is using the molecules for detection. So as part of this CBNSP program, we're designing new molecules that can detect anthrax, various other bacteria and viruses and toxins that don't have DNA. These same approaches are exactly applicable to what we're talking about today.

So what I was going to do is briefly describe how we do this, so you have an understanding of how the process works, and then I'll give you two examples of how we can apply this to anthrax. The approach is one in which we use a combination of computers and experimental methods to identify these small molecules that attach to proteins. The key here is that we're mimicking what the body does naturally when it designs and produces antibodies to attack foreign molecules that come into the bloodstream.

What makes an antibody unique is that it binds very specifically and very tightly to protein's and other molecules by making multiple contacts with them. If you can imagine trying to hold onto something, and if you hold onto something with one hand, you've got a certain amount of strength to hold the individual thing that you're attaching to, but if you have two hands or if you had multiple hands, you could hold even more tightly. That's how it works.

We use a computer to display the structure of a protein molecule. What a protein is is just a long chain of amino acids that's folded up into a ball. Upon folding, it has a surface structure that has a lot of pockets or cavities distributed across the surface.

Now the way that proteins function is by having some of these pockets interact with something else, bind to them, and then change it. What we do is we design molecules that bind into these pockets.

So the way that you can actually go about designing a very specific molecule to bind to a certain site is to use a computer to screen the hundreds of thousands of compounds that might bind to certain sites and predict which ones might, sort of rank them. Then we can go through and, instead of spending our lifetime screening 300,000, we can screen maybe 50 or 100 or 1,000 and speed up the process dramatically.

In doing that for botulinum toxin and designing molecules that bind to it, we have been able to work out the methods, so that up to 50 to 60 percent of those predicted to bind actually do bind, and that speeds up the process dramatically.

The next step, once you've identified a set of molecules that bind to one site, and then a set that bind to another site, is to link pairs of them together to give you sort of the effect of two hands, that when they attach to the protein, attach very tightly, so they don't come off, because that's what you want for an inhibitor, something that binds and doesn't leave, so it blocks the action of something else. It also gives you specificity, because it says, this one has to bind in this special site and this one has to bind in this special site, and they have to be a certain distance apart. Otherwise, they don't bind tightly.

So if you have one molecule that binds to one site and you attach another one to it, now you have this bivalent inhibitor. The two will bind on the order of a thousand to a millionfold stronger than the individual one. So that gives you the added advantage of doing this.

So the two previous examples, Dr. Smith described, and Dr. Thomas, described the production of inhibitors for furin. This is a protein where we don't know the structure of it yet, but Dr. Thomas has produced the protein and we've talked about crystallizing it, so that it's something that can be done in the near future.

The approach there would be to take known inhibitors, small molecule inhibitors for that particular protease, look at the structure of the molecule, and define another site nearby that we can target a second molecule to, that we can identify by computer modeling, and then synthesize a series of compounds that link the two together.

Now the reason we want something more specific than you currently have is that there are a lot of proteins like furins that need to function in the body. So you need to target that specific one as best you can to inhibit the activity, so that you have minimized side effects.

Now the next two examples involve a protective antigen that we've talked a lot about. One of the steps that's essential for function of the toxin, as you have seen in the model you have, is for the individual protective antigen molecules to come together to form a heptamer. Now the structural work on this, the crystal structures of these proteins have already been done. So we know what it looks like. There's actually been a fair amount of work done by others showing that there are certain regions on the surface of the protein that function by attaching each other together, where they stick together.

So one can design small molecules that target and bind around that site to block their coming together and forming protective antigen heptamers. That would be an effective set of drugs.

The next slide is a second set where you have talked about this furin protease that clips the end off the toxin, the protective antigen, so it can come together and form a heptamer. That clippage is also required for edema factor and lethal factor to attach to the top. So by designing a set of small molecules that bind to a specific site on the top of the molecule, you can actually block the toxins from being loaded on and injected into the cell.

Now these are methods that are currently being used. They have shown us that we can really speed up the process. I think that probably one really important thing to do would be, as you had asked questions before, bring together the right people, the right teams, to actually combine all of these techniques, to actually produce a series of different compounds that can be used as inhibitors. Because as, I think it was, Dr. Thomas said, what you really need is a cocktail. You don't want to rely on any one because in some cases the load is so great in these individuals by the time you've determined that they have the infection that any one probably won't work well enough.

So I think that's pretty much it.

[The prepared statement of Mr. Balhorn follows:]

Congress of the United States
House of Representatives
Committee on Government Reform

"Quickening the Pace of Research in Protecting Against Anthrax and Other Biological Terrorist Agents"

Rod Balhorn
Biology and Biotechnology Research Program
Lawrence Livermore National Laboratory

February 28, 2002

Thank you for giving me the opportunity to appear before the Committee on Government Reform to discuss the pace of research in protecting against anthrax and other biological terrorist agents. I am a biochemist employed by Lawrence Livermore National Laboratory (LLNL), a Department of Energy laboratory managed by the University of California. I commend Chairman Burton and Ranking Member Waxman for convening a hearing on what I consider an extremely important issue involving our homeland security.

As I am certain most of you recognize, the production and release of biological agents by terrorist groups or other factions has become a very real threat to the security of our Nation. We were extremely fortunate last fall that the Department of Energy, Department of Defense and other agencies had already initiated programs and begun developing the tools needed to detect and identify a variety of threat pathogens, including anthrax. It is now important for us to minimize the impact of any future anthrax exposures by quickly developing a suite of drugs that can be used in combination with vaccines or antibiotics to protect against and cure future anthrax infections.

My research group at LLNL, and my collaborators at two sister National Laboratories (Sandia National Laboratory and Brookhaven National Laboratory), have made significant advances in the development of methods needed to design and synthesize small molecules that bind to unique sites on the surfaces of proteins with high affinity and selectivity. While our current research efforts are focused entirely on producing reagents for use in threat agent detection and identification, the very same approach can and should be applied to the development of inhibitors that minimize the toxicity associated with exposures to pathogenic organisms, such as anthrax, or highly toxic proteins, such as botulinum neurotoxin.

Drug development is a well-established industry that is best carried out by biotech and pharmaceutical companies, not National Laboratories. However, in special cases of National need, such as the development of drugs that can be used to protect against future terrorist activities involving the use of biological weapons, the most rapid and efficient way to achieve the development of these compounds is by combining the efforts of scientists in our National and other governmental laboratories, Universities, National Institutes and Industry that have expertise in these areas to develop effective "lead compounds", the first and one of the most difficult steps in drug development. These "lead compounds" are the prototype molecules that exhibit the degree of inhibition desired in the final drug. The remainder of the process, which typically includes performing the metabolism, distribution and toxicity studies, clinical trials, and the optimization of synthesis and production (using conditions and materials suitable for use in humans), are best carried out by the appropriate companies in the private sector.

The speakers in Panel One have described several key steps in the progression of anthrax infections that can be targeted to design new and more effective drugs that function by blocking the cellular damage caused by the anthrax toxins. These include the initial stage of anthrax toxin activation by the protease furin and several subsequent steps that enable the toxin to enter the cell. While my group has not yet begun working on the design of anthrax toxin inhibitors, I would like to take a few minutes of your time to describe how the methods we use to design of small detection molecules at the National Laboratories could be applied to the development of a suite of new drugs that might minimize or eliminate the impact of anthrax exposures. While I will only describe two examples, these methods will be broadly applicable to other threat agents that might be produced and used by terrorist groups.

The approach mimics the method commonly used by biological molecules, such as antibodies, to bind tightly and selectively to their target by binding to multiple, neighboring sites on its surface (Figure 1). Several recent research studies have shown that two or more small molecules that normally bind to different sites on the surface of a protein with low to moderate affinities can be linked together to produce compounds that bind 100 to one million times more tightly than the original components [1-3]. While the application of this approach by others has usually been limited to linking together molecules that are known to naturally bind to the target proteins proteins (one noteable exception is the anthrax toxin inhibitor developed by Collier and Whitesides), we have discovered that a similar approach can be used to design high affinity ligands (HALs) that bind anywhere on the surface of the protein, including those that do not perform a function.

This method works because all proteins have "pockets" or cavities distributed across its surface that can be used for binding small molecules. These cavities are produced as the amino acid chain that makes up the protein is folded into a three dimensional structure to create a functional molecule (Figure 2). Our efforts to design HALs that bind to botulinum neurotoxin as part of the Chemical and Biological National Security Program, funded by the NNSA, have shown us that a combination of computational and experimental methods can be used to identify small molecules that bind with moderate affinities to unique pockets on the surface of the toxin [4]. Pairs of these molecules can be linked together using synthetic chemistry to produce HALs that only bind proteins that contain the two pockets separated by the appropriate distance (Figure 3).

The most direct approach to design these HALs uses crystal structures of the target molecules that have been determined by X-ray diffraction. Structures of the three major components of the toxin produced by the anthrax bacterium, the protective antigen, the lethal factor and the edema factor, have already been determined and are available for use. Analyses of these structures and the complexes that are formed when they combine have revealed several approaches that can be used to block the function of anthrax toxin. One has been suggested by Drs. Smith and Thomas - designing a better inhibitor to block the enzyme located on the surface of our blood cells that activates the protective antigen and initiates the formation of one active form of the toxin. This can be accomplished by crystallizing and determining the structure of this protein, called furin, and identifying a suitable small molecule that binds to a unique pocket nearby the region on the surface of the protein called the active site. A highly specific inhibitor can then be produced by linking an inhibitor, such as the one Dr. Smith has already designed to bind in the active site of furin, to the small molecule that binds to the adjacent unique pocket using synthetic chemistry (Figure 4). Inhibitors of this type would be expected to block the toxin produced by all strains of anthrax, including those that may have been changed by genetic engineering, because the target of the inhibitor is a protein located on the surface of the exposed individuals white blood cells, not a protein produced by the infecting anthrax organism.

Other approaches similar to those described by Drs. Young and Collier could be developed that block any one of several steps in the assembly of the anthrax toxin components and enable the lethal or edema factors to enter our white blood cells. In this second example, compounds would be designed to bind to one of two sites on the surface of the protective antigen. Synthetic molecules designed to bind to one site (Figure 5) would prevent the protective antigen from combining with six other molecules like itself to form a functional pore in the membrane through which the toxin passes. Other molecules could be produced that cover a second site (Figure 6) where the lethal factor attaches to the protective antigen. This would prevent the lethal factor from gaining access to the interior of the cell and eliminate its toxicity.

Clearly there are a variety of approaches that can be used to develop drugs that block the action of anthrax toxin. These drugs are most easily (and rapidly) designed once we've determined the structure of the toxin or protein target. However, other methods have been developed to identify and link together small molecules that bind to proteins with unknown structures (5). These methods require more effort and time to identify the pairs of molecules that need to be linked together to produce the inhibitors, but they offer the advantage that they can be used to design drugs that block the activity of a pathogen or protein toxin without taking the years needed to determine the structure of each target protein.

The one common feature in all these approaches is the requirement for an investment in longer-term basic research. This research is essential. We cannot design new drugs and antidotes without it. Consequently, the most effective mechanism for speeding up the pace of research in protecting against anthrax and other biological terrorist agents is to make certain that sufficient funding is earmarked for longer term (3-5 yr) basic research efforts that determine how the pathogens or other threat agents function and provide the time needed to create these new drugs and antidotes.

While our research efforts at LLNL are currently focused exclusively on designing high affinity ligands for toxin and pathogen detection (at present, no funding is being received for drug development), we have described two approaches that could utilize our same HAL design capabilities to create a suite of inhibitors that block anthrax toxin function in a relatively short (3-5 year) period of time. Such an effort, which I believe should be only one of several that are carried out, would cost ~$9 million over a five year period. While it is difficult to project how long it will take to identify suitable lead compounds, the first prototype drug candidates could be identified as early as Year 2 and a suite of several compounds that block different steps in anthrax toxin formation should be synthesized by the end of Year 4 or 5. The key elements of this effort should include the production of the furin protease by Dr. Thomas (University of Washington) and the determination of its crystal structure and the structures of protective antigen-ligand complexes, the computational analysis and computational ligand screening, and the experimental testing and identification of the ligand pairs to be linked together by various National Laboratory investigators. The synthetic chemistry might be conducted as a combined effort between Lawrence Livermore National Laboratory and Dr. Smith, an expert in furin inhibitor design. Upon completion of the initial testing of a set of lead compounds, a suitable industrial partner would be identified, using procedures already established by the Department of Energy and the University of California, to license and complete the testing and eventual production of the final drugs.

References:

1. 1. Shuker, S.B., Hajduk, P.J., Meadows, R.P. and Fesik, S.W. (1996) Discovering High Affinity Ligands for Proteins: SAR by NMR. Science 274: 1531-4.
2. Kramer, R.H. and Karpen, J.W. (1998) Spanning Binding Sites on Allosteric Proteins with Polymer-linked Ligand Dimers. Nature 395: 710-3.
3. Fan, E., Merritt, E.A., Verlinde, C.L. and Hol W.G. (2000) AB(5) Toxins: Structures and Inhibitor Design. Curr. Opin. Struct. Biol. 10: 680-6.
4. Lightstone, F.C., Prieto, M.C., Singh, A.K., Piqueras, M.C., Whittal, R.M., Knapp, M.S., Balhorn,R. and Roe, D.C. (2000) The Identification of Novel Small Molecule Ligands that Bind to Tetanus Toxin. Chemical Research Toxicology 13, 356-362.

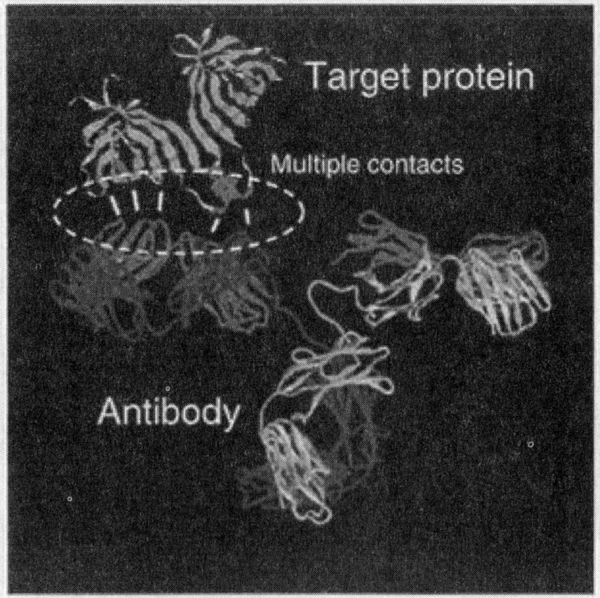

Figure 1. The multiple contacts that occur between antibodies and the proteins they target lead to the antibody's high affinity and selectivity.

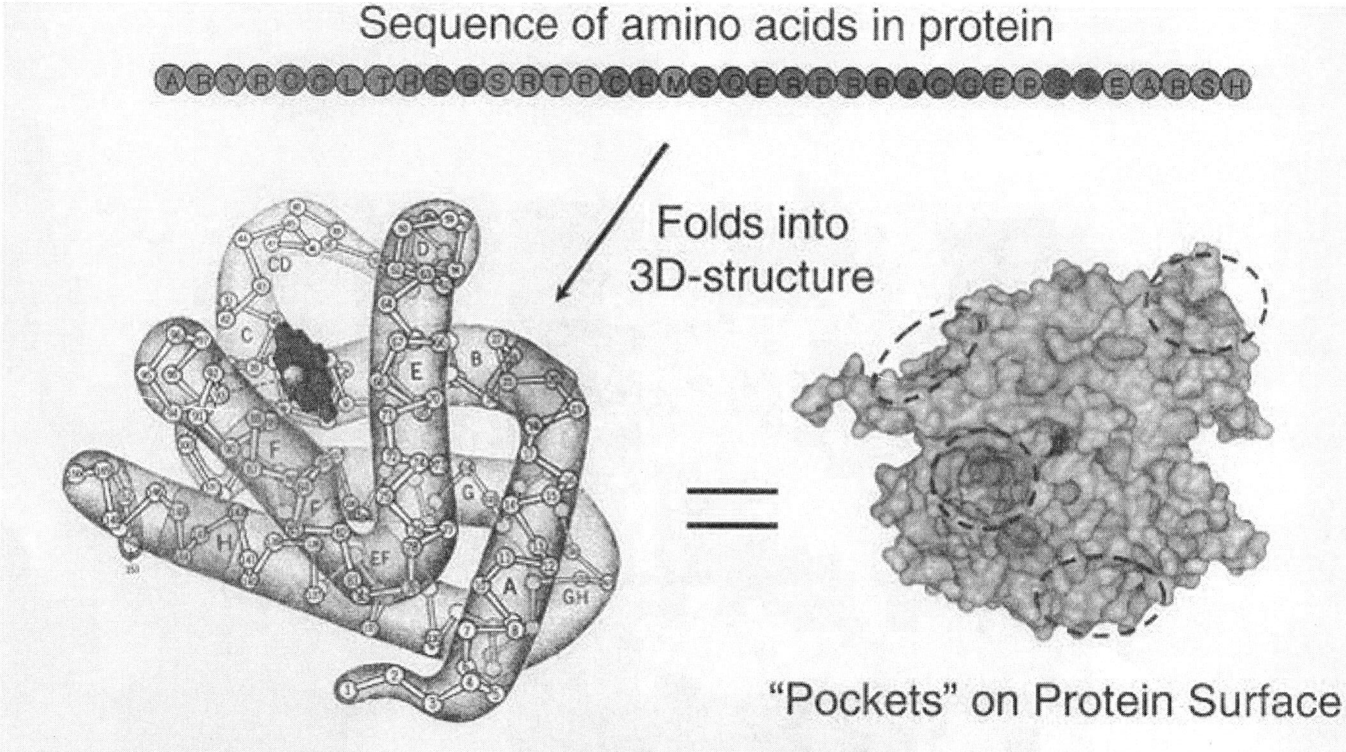

Figure 2. Proteins, which are a folded chain of amino acids, have "pockets" or cavities distributed all over their surface.

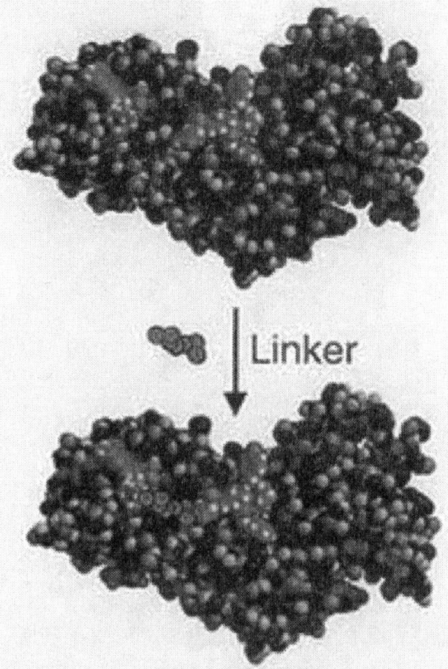

Figure 3. High affinity ligands that bind to specific sites on the surfaces of proteins can be created by linking together pairs of weaker-binding ligands that bind to two or more neighboring sites.

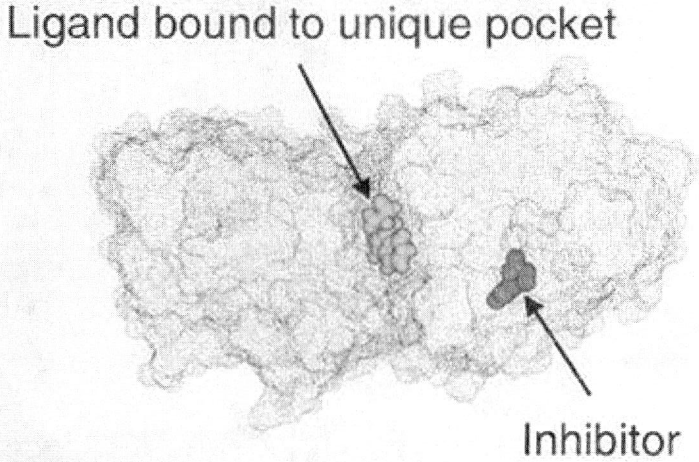

Figure 4. Furin inhibitors with increased selectivity can be produced by linking together existing inhibitors that bind in the active site (red) and small molecules (yellow) identified to bind to unique sites nearby.

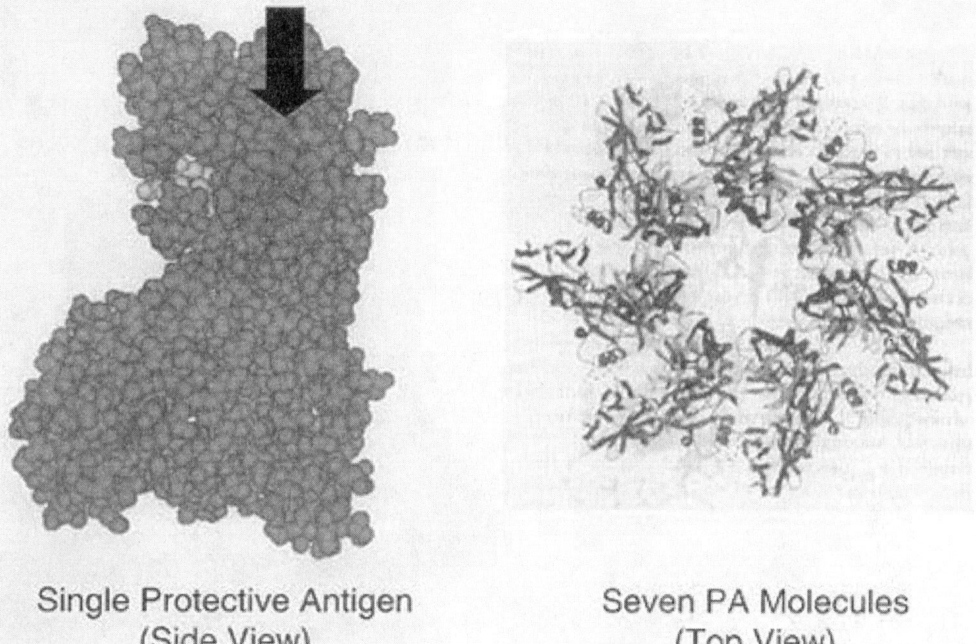

Figure 5. High affinity ligands designed to bind to a site (red) on the Protective Antigen that enables the linking of seven Protective Antigen molecules together on the cell's surface (right, view from top) could be used to block the formation of functional toxin

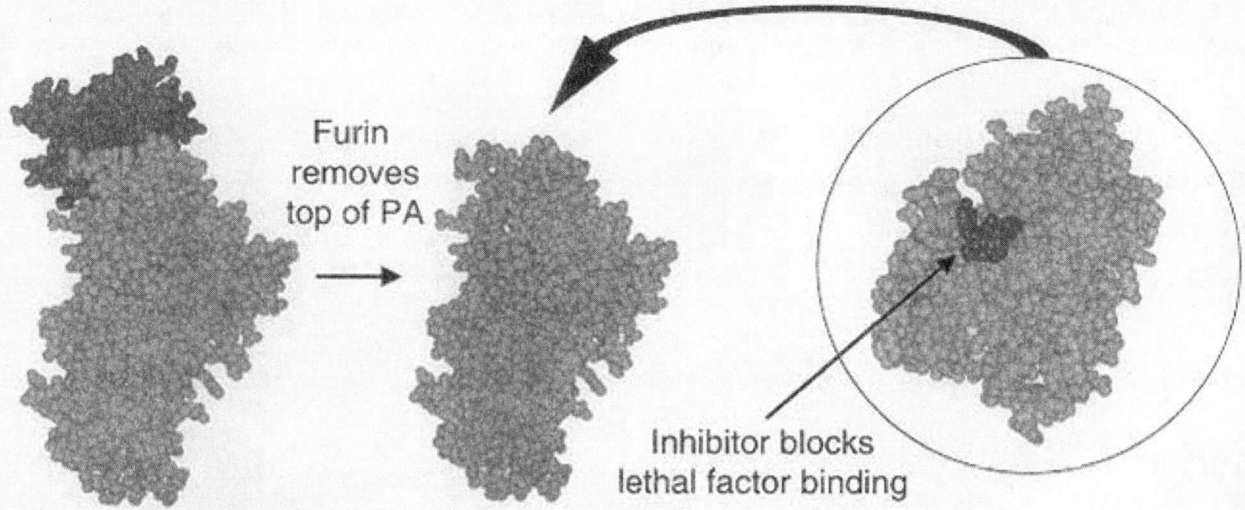

Figure 6. Removal of one end of the Protective Antigen following cleavage by the Furin allows the Lethal Factor to bind to PA. Inhibitors could be designed to block the ability of the Lethal Factor to bind to PA.

Mr. BURTON. We'll get back to you with questions.

Dr. Leppla.

Mr. LEPPLA. Mr. Chairman, members of the committee, I appreciate the opportunity to appear before you today to describe my research regarding anthrax toxin and the role of the protease furin in anthrax toxin action. Included in my remarks will be some discussion about the possible use of furin inhibitors to block anthrax toxin action and the potential this holds for treatment of anthrax infections.

Also here today is Dr. Carole Heilman. Dr. Heilman is the Director of the Division of Microbiology and Infectious Diseases of the National Institute of Allergy and Infectious Diseases. As you know, the NIAID spearheads the bioterrorism research effort at the National Institutes of Health, and in fact the NIAID supported the recent studies by Drs. Collier and Young which we've heard described today, which has elucidated important aspects of the mechanism by which anthrax toxin destroys cells. As we've heard, the information gained from these NIH-supported studies is likely to hasten development of new drugs to treat anthrax. Dr. Heilman will be pleased to respond to questions you may have regarding NIAID efforts to counter bioterrorism.

First, in regard to my own work, I have some comments in my written testimony regarding work that I have done in previous years on the anthrax toxin receptors. I think I'll just abbreviate that because you've heard the elegant work done by Dr. Young, which identified the anthrax toxin receptor, and that work was published in Nature several months ago. It showed that the anthrax toxin receptor is, indeed, probably this molecule called tumor endothelial marker 8. That protein was, in fact, described just 1 year ago by Dr. Ken Kinzler at Johns Hopkins University, and that's, of course, work supported by the National Cancer Institute.

So as Drs. Young and Collier pointed out in their publication, as was mentioned earlier, their discovery opens several avenues toward development of new therapies. Specifically, they showed that a portion of the receptor, essentially a receptor decoy made in Escherichia coli, was able to block toxin action in cultured cells. There's good precedent for receptor decoys being effective therapeutic agents. There's a drug on the market called Enbrel, which is a tumor necrosis factor soluble receptor. It is a decoy, and it is quite effective in treating rheumatoid arthritis. So there's good precedent for the approach that they have described.

Then I can also refer to some of my own work on furin. You've heard this protein described. Furin is a member of a family of similar enzymes that are required for generating the final active forms of hormones such as insulin. It's an essential enzyme, as was mentioned by Dr. Thomas. There's what's called the "mouse knockout." That is, if you knock out the gene in mice, that causes the death of mice during embryonic development. So that does show that the enzyme furin is an essential enzyme.

I began work on anthrax toxin a number of years ago. At that time it was clear that a number of bacterial toxins require proteolytic activation. That is, the toxins had to be cut at a specific site to be made fully active.

During our first efforts to purify anthrax toxin protective antigen, we recognized that it was very easily cleaved at a single site by cellular proteases and by bacterial proteases. We identified the cleavage site to be a sequence of four amino acids: arginine-lysine-lysine-arginine. We then showed that removal of that cleavage site by changing the protein made anthrax toxin inactive. So this was proof that cleavage at that site was absolutely required for the toxin to be effective.

We set out to identify the cellular protease that was required for anthrax toxin action. We did this by changing a small number of amino acids within the protein sequence of protective antigen by a mutagenesis procedure, and we replaced each of the amino acids in this sequence arg-lys-lys-arg, which we had defined as the point at which cleavage occurred.

We found that any toxin that had arginine at both the first and the fourth positions was toxic to cells. It didn't matter what was in the second and third positions.

At the time that we were doing this work, other researchers, as you have heard, had been looking for many years and finally had found this family of proteases, of which furin is a member, because these are essential enzymes required to process proteins like the insulin precursor. Persons working in that field had identified one member of that family, the protease we've heard a lot about, furin, and, in fact, suggested that the sequence that it recognized was exactly the same as what we had defined in the anthrax toxin protein. So we suggested that anthrax toxin was being cleaved by furin, and we began a collaboration with Gary Thomas, which you've heard about. He quickly proved that purified furin does, indeed, cleave protective antigen.

Subsequently, we generated mutated cultured cells. This is a very convenient model system. We made these cells, which lack functional furin, and we showed that these cells were highly resistant to anthrax toxin and other toxins. In fact, similar mutant cells had been made earlier by Thomas Moehring at the University of Vermont, but the genetic defect in the cells wasn't known at that point.

We showed that the furin-deficient cells were resistant to several toxins. Dr. Moehring had already shown that these cells are also resistant to a number of viruses. It's been mentioned that furin is required for viral envelope protein activation.

My lab has actually not been working actively on furin in the last few years, although we're beginning again to do this, but, as you've heard, Dr. Thomas has continued to work actively and productively in that field. He's provided us a full account of the important role of furin.

So now I want to offer some comments regarding possible therapeutic opportunities for anthrax infections. As was mentioned, we've identified at least eight stages which the toxin must pass through in order to achieve its ultimate killing action on cells. Studies in cell structure models have demonstrated the principle that each of these stages can be blocked, and Drs. Collier, Young and Friedlander from USAMRIID have provided much of the data showing that each of these separate stages represents a valid target to which we could point therapeutic interventions.

In trying to find targets for intervening in infectious diseases, most researchers will focus on identifying target molecules that are unique to the pathogen. In the case of anthrax, a unique target is the anthrax toxin lethal factor. It's been shown that Bacillus anthracis bacteria lacking lethal factor are greatly weakened in their ability to cause disease. As we've heard, there's the precedent of treating HIV with protease inhibitors, so I think there are many researchers who believe that there's a great opportunity for the treatment of anthrax by using and developing inhibitors of lethal factor protease. Pharmaceutical companies and academic researchers have extensive experience in developing inhibitors of proteases, and already some of that expertise is being redirected toward developing lethal factor inhibitors.

The NIAID has for several years been supporting at least two research groups studying lethal factor structure and inhibitor development. An important advance in this area occurred several months ago with the publication of the crystal structure of the lethal factor protease. This work was done in the laboratory of Robert Liddington at the Burnham Institute in La Jolla, CA. Dr. Collier and I were collaborators in that work.

The availability of the complete crystal structure of lethal factor has encouraged many researchers to either begin or intensify existing efforts to develop lethal factor inhibitors. My lab is providing purified lethal factor protein to a number of these groups to facilitate their work. I personally have considerable hope that this developmental effort will lead to a specific lethal factor inhibitor that, in fact, will have efficacy in treatment of anthrax.

The other protease, of course, involved in anthrax toxin action is furin, which we've heard about. I can abbreviate my comments here. In addition to the inhibitor that Dr. Thomas has developed, which is to my knowledge the most potent furin inhibitor available, which I know by the names of the "Portland" inhibitor or the PDX inhibitor, potent furin inhibitors have also been developed by two other NIH-funded researchers, Drs. Iris Lindberg, of Louisiana State University, and Robert Fuller, of the University of Michigan. The inhibitors developed by these three NIH-funded researchers, now including Dr. Thomas, employ three different approaches to inhibitor design, and together identify a number of opportunities for development of even more potent furin inhibitors.

It should be mentioned that intramural NIH researchers have also made important contributions in regard to furin research. Drs. David FitzGerald and Ira Pastan of the National Cancer Institute proved that furin has an essential role in the activation of Pseudomonas exotoxin. Dr. Juan Bonifacino of the National Institute of Child Health and Human Development has provided important knowledge about the movement of furin between various compartments within a cell. Several other NIH-funded studies include analysis of the properties and functions of furin as a part of larger studies of various disease processes. This portfolio of investigator-initiated extramural and intramural research provides a strong knowledge base on which to base therapies for those diseases in which furin plays a role.

I mentioned earlier that drug developers prefer to target molecules that are unique to a pathogen. For this reason, I think furin has received less attention as a target for drug development. The expectation has been that inhibition of this enzyme, which plays an essential role in many normal processes, might cause significant physiological damage to normal tissue. Consistent with that prediction is the fact I mentioned before, that genetic inactivation of furin causes death of mouse embryos. Nevertheless, I do believe that inhibition of furin should be examined as one possible avenue toward development of therapies for anthrax. I'm encouraged by Dr. Thomas' remarks regarding the preliminary toxicity studies of his inhibitor that perhaps current inhibitors may not be as toxic as one might predict.

Given the renewed interest in anthrax, I anticipate that the furin inhibitors mentioned above, as well as others, will be evaluated for anthrax toxin inhibition in appropriate cell culture models in the near future, and if they're successful, we hope they will be carried forward to clinical use.

That concludes my testimony.

[The prepared statement of Mr. Leppla follows:]

Testimony
Before the Committee on Government Reform
United States House of Representatives

Quickening the Pace of Research In Protecting Against Anthrax and Other Biological Terrorist Agents–A Look at Toxin Interference

Statement of
Stephen Leppla, Ph.D.
Senior Investigator, Oral Infection and Immunity Branch, Division of Intramural Research, National Institute of Dental and Craniofacial Research, National Institutes of Health

For Release on Delivery
February 28, 2002

Mr. Chairman and Members of the Committee:

I appreciate the opportunity to appear before you today to describe my research regarding anthrax toxin receptors and the role of the protease furin in anthrax toxin action. Included in my remarks will be some discussion about the possible use of furin inhibitors to block anthrax toxin action, and the potential this holds for the treatment of anthrax infections.

The National Institute of Allergy and Infectious Diseases (NIAID) spearheads the bioterrorism research effort at the National Institutes of Heath (NIH) and supported the recent studies by Dr. John Collier, Harvard University, and Dr. John Young, University of Wisconsin Medical School, who are present today, which elucidated the mechanisms by which anthrax toxin destroys cells. The information gained through these studies will likely hasten the development of new drugs to treat anthrax.

NIAID also supports a number of other drug development efforts for anthrax and other Category A agents of bioterrorism. Earlier in the month, NIAID sponsored a Blue Ribbon Panel on Bioterrorism and its Implications for Biomedical Research, which brought together a distinguished panel of leaders from the biomedical research community and experts in Category A agents of bioterrorism to obtain expert advice and input on NIAID's Counter-Bioterrorism Research Agenda. This group helped NIAID assess its current research efforts to counter bioterrorism and identified goals for NIAID to implement on an immediate and intermediate/long-term basis. Indeed, one of the immediate goals identified for anthrax research is to encourage exploration of new targets for antimicrobial therapies, including strategies to prevent germination of spores, the synthesis or neutralization of toxins, and interference with attachment and entry of toxins into host target cells, which will build upon the findings of Drs. Young and Collier.

First I wish to briefly discuss our work on the cellular receptor for anthrax toxin. Bacterial toxins that attack animal cells must first bind to the surface of those cells. Several toxins do this by interacting with a single specific protein present on the cell surface. By definition, this protein is the toxin receptor. The receptor is typically a normal cellular protein that has a recognized role in cell function. It is only by accident that this protein is used by a bacterial toxin to enter the cell and damage it. I began studies intended to identify the anthrax toxin receptor some years ago while a researcher at the United States Army Medical Research Institute of Infectious Diseases (USAMRIID) in Frederick, MD, and continued this work after transferring to the National Institute of Dental and Craniofacial Research (NIDCR) in 1989. Our early work showed that all types of cells have anthrax toxin receptors, that cells typically have about 10,000 receptor molecules on their surface, and that the receptors were probably proteins. We generated cultured cell mutants lacking functional anthrax toxin receptors. Over a period of years, we worked intermittently to identify the receptor, using various biochemical and genetic methods, but our efforts were unsuccessful. Several years ago, a group at Harvard University began similar efforts, and they were successful in identifying the receptor last summer. This work, led by Drs. John Young and John Collier and supported by the NIAID, was published in the journal *Nature* several months ago. This important work showed that anthrax toxin uses as its receptor a protein named tumor endothelial marker 8, or TEM8. This cell surface protein had been described just one year ago in work from the laboratory of Dr. Ken Kinzler of Johns Hopkins University, work supported by the National Cancer Institute. The protein was identified as one that is highly expressed in tumor endothelial cells.

As Drs. Young and Collier pointed out in their publication, and as I mentioned earlier, their important discovery opens potential several avenues toward development of new therapies for anthrax infection.

Specifically, they showed that a portion of the receptor, produced as a recombinant protein in the common bacterium *Esherichia coli*, was able to act as a receptor decoy and block the action of toxin in cultured cells. A precedent for receptor decoys being effective therapeutic agents is provided by the tumor necrosis factor soluble receptor, marketed as the product Enbrel, which is used in treating rheumatoid arthritis.

Now let me turn to describing work performed in my own laboratory on furin. Furin is a cellular protease which is required for the processing of many proteins that a cell secretes or delivers to its cell surface. Furin is a member of a family of similar enzymes that include those required for generating the final, active forms of peptide hormones such as insulin. It is an essential enzyme, as indicated by the fact that inactivation of the gene in mice causes death during an early stage of embryonic development.

When I began work on anthrax toxin, there were already several examples of bacterial toxins that require proteolytic activation. That is, the toxins had to be cut at a specific site by a protease enzyme to be made fully active. During our first efforts to purify the protective antigen protein of anthrax toxin, we noted that it was very easily cleaved by proteases at a single site. By sequence analysis of the fragments, we determined that the protein was cleaved following a sequence of four amino acids, arginine-lysine-lysine-arginine. We then showed that removal of this cleavage site inactivated the toxin. This was convincing proof that cleavage at this site is essential for anthrax toxin action. Because uncleaved toxin was fully active when added to cells, we suspected that the cells were causing proteolytic activation of the toxin. In effect, the toxin appeared to be using a cellular protease to achieve its own activation.

We then set out to identify the cellular protease required for anthrax toxin activation. We changed the amino acids within the arginine-lysine-lysine-arginine sequence, replacing each amino acid with many different ones. By comparing the toxicity of more than 30 mutated proteins, we found that any toxin protein having arginine at both the first and fourth positions was toxic to cells. The identity of the amino acids in the two middle positions occupied by lysine in the original sequence could be changed to other amino acids with little effect. At the time this work was being done, other researchers had finally identified the long-sought human proteases which process biosynthetic precursors of hormones such as insulin. It had been thought that these proteases recognize only paired basic amino acid residues such as the sequence arginine-arginine. However, the new evidence suggested that one of these proteases, named furin, cleaves proteins having arginines at the first and fourth positions. Because this sequence exactly matched the one we had identified, we speculated that furin was the cellular protease that was needed to activate anthrax toxin protective antigen. We then contacted Dr. Gary Thomas, of the Vollum Institute, University of Oregon. Dr. Thomas was already a recognized expert in study of these cellular proteases, and he agreed to collaborate in further studies. He quickly determined that purified fur rapidly cleaves the anthrax toxin protective antigen protein.

Subsequently, we generated mutated cultured cells lacking functional furin, and showed that these were highly resistant to anthrax toxin. Similar mutant cells had been produced some years earlier by Thomas Moehring, University of Vermont, but the genetic defect in the cells was not known. We went on to show that the furin-deficient cells are also resistant to several other bacterial proteins that require protease activation, and Dr. Moehring had already shown that such cells are resistant to certain viruses. In was later shown through work in other laboratories that furin is involved in the activation of many viral envelope proteins, including those of influenza virus and HIV. My lab has not been actively working on furin in the last several years, although we continue to aid others investigators in this field by supplying the furin-deficient cultured cells when requested. My original collaborator in the furin studies, Dr. Gary Thomas, has continued to work actively and productively in this field, and he can provide details about the current state of research on furin.

I now would like to offer some comments comparing possible therapeutic opportunities for anthrax infections. Researchers working on anthrax have identified at least eight distinct stages at which one theoretically could interfere with anthrax toxin action. Studies in cell culture models have demonstrated in principle that each of these stages can be blocked. Drs. Collier, Young, and Dr. Arthur Friedlander, USAMRIID, have provided much of the data proving that these separate stages each represent a target for therapeutic interventions.

In trying to find targets for therapeutic intervention in infectious diseases, most researchers focus on identifying target molecules that are unique to the pathogen. For example, one attractive target is the anthrax toxin lethal factor. *Bacillus anthracis* bacteria lacking lethal factor are greatly weakened in their ability to cause anthrax. Because of the success with which AIDS is treated by inhibitors of the HIV viral protease, many researchers believe that there is a great opportunity for treatment of anthrax with inhibitors of the lethal factor protease. Pharmaceutical companies and academic researchers have extensive experience in developing inhibitors of proteases, and some of that expertise is being redirected toward developing lethal factor inhibitors. NIAID has for several years been supporting at least two research groups studying lethal factor structure and inhibitor development. An important advance in this area occurred several months ago with the publication of the crystal structure of the lethal factor protease, work done in the laboratory of Robert Liddington, Burnham Institute, La Jolla, CA. Dr.

Collier and I were collaborators in that work. The availability of the complete crystal structure of lethal factor has encouraged many researchers to begin new efforts or intensify existing efforts to develop lethal factor inhibitors. My lab is providing purified lethal factor protein to several of these groups so as to facilitate their work. I have considerable hope that a carefully selected lethal factor inhibitor will prove to be an effective therapeutic for anthrax.

The other protease involved in anthrax toxin action is the one discussed above, the cellular protease furin. Because of the important role furin has in normal physiological processes, NIH has supported many studies involving furin and the family of proteases which are closely related to it. For example, NIH has supported the work of Dr. Thomas over a number of years, during which time he developed the potent inhibitor which he calls the "Portland" inhibitor. Potent furin inhibitors have also been developed by two other NIH-funded researchers, Drs. Iris Lindberg, of Louisana State University, and Robert Fuller, of the University of Michigan. The inhibitors developed by these three NIH-funded researchers employ three different approaches to inhibitor design, and together identify a number of opportunities for development of even more potent furin inhibitors. It should be mentioned that NIH intramural researchers have also made important contributions in furin research. Drs. David FitzGerald and Ira Pastan of the National Cancer Institute proved that furin has an essential role in the action of *Pseudomonas* exotoxin. Dr. Juan Bonifacino of the National Institute of Child Health and Human Development has provided important knowledge about the movement of furin between various compartments within a cell. Several other NIH-funded studies include analysis of the properties and functions of furin as a part of larger studies of various disease processes. This portfolio of investigator-initiated extramural and intramural research is producing a strong knowledge base on which to base therapies for those diseases in which furin plays a role.

I mentioned earlier that drug developers prefer to target molecules that are unique to a pathogen. For this reason, furin has received less attention as a target for drug development. The expectation has been that inhibition of this enzyme, which plays an essential role in many normal processes, might cause significant physiological damage to normal tissue. Consistent with that prediction is the fact mentioned above, that genetic inactivation of furin causes death of mouse embryos. Nevertheless, I do believe that inhibition of furin should be examined as one possible therapy for anthrax. Given the renewed interest in anthrax, I anticipate that the furin inhibitors mentioned above, as well as others, will be evaluated for anthrax toxin inhibition in appropriate cell culture models in the near future.

That concludes my testimony. I would be happy to respond to any questions that you or Members of the Committee may have.

Mr. BURTON. Thank you very much, Doctor.

We will now hear from Dr. Friedlander.

Dr. FRIEDLANDER. Mr. Chairman, it's a privilege to appear before the committee today on my very last day of active duty in the U.S. Army.

[Applause.]

Mr. BURTON. We hope you are going to stay on as a consultant.

Dr. FRIEDLANDER. I'm planning to.

I welcome the opportunity to explain my published remarks on the approaches to managing anthrax bioterrorist attacks. I am here to discuss the scientific issues. Other questions dealing with the DOD's research portfolio, the funding, and policy have been forwarded to OSD, and they are preparing a response for the committee.

I am a physician trained in infectious diseases and a scientist who has worked in research in infectious diseases, including anthrax, for many years. The effective management of human cases of anthrax is dependent upon our knowledge both of the bacterium that causes this disease as well as the processes by which the bacterium counteracts the normal host defense mechanisms.

Anthrax is due to the invasion and prolific growth of the bacterium in host organs and the production of toxins and other disease-enhancing factors. Thus, anthrax is, like other diseases, caused by invasive bacteria such as the pneumococcus, the streptococcus, and those causing serious hospital-acquired infections. It is distinctly unlike bacteria that cause disease solely by their production of toxins without invading the host, such as diphtheria, tetanus, and botulism.

Inhalational anthrax begins and is concentrated in the central portion of the chest, where it destroys the tissue architecture. This leads to large accumulations of fluid, often with blood in it, in and around the lung, and this is an important contributor to the cause of death.

The toxins are thought to be harmful to the body's phagocytic cells that are normally responsible for destroying the bacteria when it comes in. The toxins may also cause the release of chemical mediators from host cells that, in turn, when they are present in excess, can contribute directly to death of the host.

Now there are three general ways that we deal with infectious diseases such as anthrax. The first is prevention of the disease by vaccination. The second is destruction of the bacterium by antibiotics, and the third is neutralization of the organism's toxins or the toxin-induced chemical mediators that contribute to disease.

Now prevention of disease with vaccination is the ideal because any invasive bacterial disease, including anthrax, has a high mortality. The mainstay of treatment for this disease, anthrax, as for other invasive bacteria infections, is antibiotics. Antibiotic treatment, coupled with modern clinical management in the current outbreak, has established that although the disease is not invariably fatal, nonetheless, mortality remains high.

Effective treatment of anthrax has been demonstrated, however, only with a very limited number of antibiotics, but in the test tube the organism is susceptible to many antibiotics that have not yet been tested for their efficacy.

Now knowledge of the toxins has developed over the last 20 years with very significant and important advances being made in the last few years. The committee has heard about these in-depth from the previous presenters, and I won't repeat these statements, but my comments are present in my written testimony.

In theory, as has been suggested, it should be possible to develop rational anti-toxin treatments that target each and every of the at least eight steps in the intoxication process, from the initial binding to the damage to the cell. We've heard about non-toxic mutant PA molecules and small molecule inhibitors and the soluble toxin receptor that had been shown to neutralize the toxin, and it's anticipated that others targeting various pathways will be found.

Other approaches, however, to anti-toxin therapy might focus on developing treatments that neutralize those chemical mediators that are released from the cell when the toxin damages the cell. In fact, there have been decades of research that has only recently led to the licensure of such a drug that counteracts the effects of mediators produced during other invasive bacterial infections. This drug is now licensed, and similar approaches should be taken with anthrax. It's likely, however, that as with other invasive bacterial infections, these anti-toxin treatments will be used as adjunctive therapy to antibiotics.

A final therapeutic approach is based upon the use of antibodies against the toxin and the bacterium. Antibodies were used in the pre-antibiotic era to treat human cases of anthrax, and animal experiments suggest they are of some value. In fact, attempts to develop human antibodies against the toxin are under development as adjunctive therapies.

In summary, then, prevention of infection remains the ideal, and antibiotics constitute the mainstay of treatment. New antibiotics, as well as adjunctive therapies to include the wide possibilities with anti-toxins and antibodies, all need to be evaluated rapidly in carefully controlled studies.

Now because of the difficulty of performing human trials, the testing of new antibiotics and adjunctive therapies will require the development of a large-scale capability for carrying out such studies in the appropriate animal models.

That's the end of my testimony.

[The prepared statement of Dr. Friedlander follows:]

Written Testimony for presentation on 28 February 2002 to the House Committee on Government Reform

Arthur M. Friedlander, M.D.

Colonel, MC

Senior Military Scientist

U. S. Army Medical Research Institute of Infectious Diseases

The effective management of human cases of anthrax is dependent upon our knowledge of both the bacterium itself and the pathogenesis of the disease, that is, the processes by which the organism overcomes the body's natural defense mechanisms.

Anthrax infection is due to the invasion and subsequent prolific growth of the bacterium in host organs and the production of the toxins and other disease enhancing factors such as the capsular material surrounding the bacterium. Additional factors contributing to the disease process remain to be discovered. Thus, anthrax is like other diseases caused by invasive bacterial organisms that may result in sepsis, such as the pneumococcus, the streptococcus, and those causing serious hospital acquired infections. Anthrax is distinctly unlike the bacterial diseases that cause disease solely by their production of toxins, such as diphtheria, tetanus, and botulism. The anthrax organism invades essentially all organs, growing to very high levels. The infection begins and is concentrated in the central portion of the chest where it destroys the tissue architecture, and is thought to obstruct normal blood and lymph flow. This leads to large accumulations of fluid, often with hemorrhage, in and around the lungs, which are important factors in the mechanism of death. Pathological examination of the tissues of human cases supports the suggestion that mechanical factors and direct damage to blood vessels are among the major causes of death.

The anthrax toxins are thought to be harmful to host phagocytic cells that are normally responsible for killing bacteria, although much remains to be established conclusively. The toxins likely have their effect early in the infectious process at the site of initial bacterial growth. Very late in the infection, when there are very high levels of bacteria in the blood, the toxins are also present in large amounts in the blood. The toxins may also cause release of chemical mediators from the host cells that, when present in excess, can directly contribute to death of the host. However, the actual mechanism of death remains to be firmly established.

There are three general ways to deal with infectious diseases such as anthrax. The first is prevention of the disease by vaccination. The second is destruction of the bacterium by antibiotics and the third is treatment to neutralize the organism's toxins or the excessive amount of toxin-induced chemical mediators that may contribute to disease.

Prevention of disease with vaccination is the ideal because any invasive bacterial disease, particularly anthrax, is associated with a high mortality even using modern treatment regimens. Effective treatment requires early recognition of the infection. The mainstay of treatment for anthrax, as for other invasive bacterial infections, is antibiotics. It is necessary to rapidly inhibit the growth and destroy the organism. Antibiotic treatment of anthrax infection coupled with modern clinical management has established that the disease is not invariably fatal, in agreement with some previous animal work. Nonetheless, mortality remains high as it is in sepsis due to other bacteria. Effective treatment of anthrax in humans or animals has been demonstrated with only a limited number of antibiotics. However, in the test tube, the bacterium is susceptible to many antibiotics that have yet to be evaluated for efficacy in either humans or animal models.

Knowledge of the anthrax toxins has been developed over the last 20 years with several new significant advances being made in the last few years. This will help in the rational development of anti-toxin treatments. The two anthrax toxins are comprised of three proteins, a cell receptor binding protein, protective antigen (PA), and two enzymes, lethal factor (LF), a zinc containing protease, and edema factor (EF), an adenylate cyclase. PA combined with LF constitutes lethal toxin; PA combined with EF comprises edema toxin. In cell culture studies, PA binds to a specific cell receptor, is activated by a cell-surface protease and converted to a heptamer (seven PA molecules), and subsequently binds either LF or EF (or both). The complex of PA and LF or EF then passes into the cell interior to exert its toxicity and damage the cell, thus interfering with its ability to counteract the anthrax bacterium. Several features of this model remain to be established. In addition to the cell-surface protease, a serum protease is capable of cleaving PA, and complexes of PA with LF occur in the serum of infected animals. The relative importance of the two proteases in toxin action *in vivo* is unknown. In summary, the toxin binds to a host cell, is activated by a host protease and then enters the cell and damages it.

Several recent findings have extended our knowledge about the toxins. This includes reports on the detailed crystal structure of both LF and EF, to go along with that previously described for PA; the identification of the cell surface receptor for PA; and the description of a cellular protein responsible for resistance to the toxic effects of LF.

These research findings have suggested various ways in which it may be possible to develop anti-toxin treatments that neutralize the damaging effects of the toxins on the cells of the host. In theory, it should be possible to develop anti-toxin treatments that target each one of the discrete steps in the intoxication process, from the initial binding to the cell, to the protease activation and various subsequent steps leading to cell damage. Indeed, non-toxic mutant PA molecules that interfere with transfer of the toxin inside the cell as well as small molecules that block the binding of LF or EF to PA have been discovered. In laboratory studies, these molecules can neutralize the damaging effect of the toxin.

Identification of the cellular receptor for PA has added greatly to our understanding of the toxins. Future therapies to neutralize toxin may include use of soluble toxin receptors and inhibitors of PA binding. Further attempts to block the toxin activating protease and the direct enzymatic activities of the toxins may also lead to effective anti-toxin treatments. For all the potential anti-toxin therapies, detailed knowledge of toxin kinetics during infection will be required, as the timing for delivery of therapeutics is critical. Anti-toxins may need to be present early in the infection before toxins become fixed to cells.

Another approach to anti-toxin therapy might focus on developing molecules that protect the cell from the damage produced by the toxin, rather than blocking the toxin itself. In addition, as noted above, it is possible that the harmful effects of the toxin are due to release of chemical mediators from the cell that act to damage other body organs. Decades of research have been devoted to counteracting such mediators produced during sepsis associated with other bacterial infections. The recent licensure of such a drug to counteract the downstream mediators of sepsis associated with other invasive bacterial infections, suggests that similar adjunctive therapies should be studied in anthrax. It is likely however, as with other invasive bacterial infections, that anti-toxin treatments of anthrax will be used as adjunctive therapy to antibiotics.

A final therapeutic approach is based upon the use of antibodies against the toxin and the bacterium itself. Antibodies were used to treat humans with anthrax in the pre-antibiotic era and animal experiments suggest they are of some value in counteracting the infection as well as the toxin. It is known that antibodies can be developed that are effective anti-toxins, in that they neutralize the effect of the toxins, as do the non-antibody anti-toxins described above. Antibodies can also be developed against other components of the bacterium and so may have multiple sites of action. Attempts to develop human antibodies to the toxin are under development as adjunctive therapy.

In summary, prevention of infection remains the ideal, and antibiotics constitute the mainstay of treatment. New antibiotics as well as adjunctive therapies to include anti-toxins, anti-sepsis mediators and antibodies all need to be evaluated in carefully controlled studies. Because of the difficulty of performing human trials, the testing of new antibiotics and adjunctive therapies will require the development of a large-scale capability for carrying out such studies in appropriate animal models.

Dr. WELDON [assuming Chair]. Thank you very much. I enjoyed all of your testimony.

Dr. Friedlander, I understand the protective antigen was labeled as a protective antigen because it produces protective antibodies in the bloodstream.

Dr. FRIEDLANDER. That's correct.

Dr. WELDON. It can't be the only protective antibody in the bloodstream. The vaccine, I'm just kind of curious how that would prevent the proliferation of the bacterial infection antibodies against the protective antigen. Can you explain that to me?

Dr. FRIEDLANDER. I'll try. As Dr. Young mentioned, there's a lot we don't know about this infection. There's a lot we don't know about how the vaccine protects.

We do know that I think most people believe that the predominant component that is protected, and it's been demonstrated with highly purified protein, is protected antigen.

Dr. WELDON. But protective antigen is sort of an endotoxin that's released——

Dr. FRIEDLANDER. Correct, an exotoxin.

Dr. WELDON. Exotoxin——

Dr. FRIEDLANDER. Right.

Dr. WELDON [continuing]. That is released by the bacteria. So if I have antibodies to protective antigen, how do they prevent the bacteria from proliferating in my lungs and in the lymph nodes in my pulmonary hylum?

Dr. FRIEDLANDER. First of all——

Dr. WELDON. You don't know, correct?

Dr. FRIEDLANDER. We don't know for sure. We do know a few things, and I'll just briefly mention them.

First of all, there is some proliferation that occurs, even in a protected animal, as is the case with other vaccines. It's not necessarily a sterile immunity.

Second, the antibodies that are produced do neutralize the toxin, but, in addition, they appear to have some effect on the bacterium itself. This is an area that is being actively pursued.

Dr. WELDON. The current vaccine that is available right now, what is in that vaccine?

Dr. FRIEDLANDER. I know that there is protective antigen in there, and it's reported that there are small amounts of the lethal factor as well.

Dr. WELDON. OK.

Dr. FRIEDLANDER. I don't know the actual composition.

Dr. WELDON. Very good.

Both of you gentlemen encouraged the further research for the development of these drugs that can be used against the toxins. In the first panel, during the questioning, I mentioned that I saw this as being complementary, and I think you made this statement very eloquently, Dr. Friedlander, in managing these diseases. As I understand it, the current drug that's on the market for treating septic shock, the one that was just released——

Dr. FRIEDLANDER. Yes.

Dr. WELDON [continuing]. What is the name of that product?

Dr. FRIEDLANDER. It's activated protein C.

Dr. WELDON. Activated protein C. That's fairly expensive, correct?

Dr. FRIEDLANDER. I'm not sure what the cost is.

Dr. WELDON. You're not sure? One of the issues that will come into play in its clinical application is, does the patient really need it, because of the huge amount of cost associated with administering it. Do you see that as a hurdle for the application of some of the technologies you're developing right now for the development of these products?

Dr. FRIEDLANDER. I think it is. As was alluded to before, I think in the first panel, one of the problems with developing very narrowly focused therapeutics is the marketplace, and that's difficult to support other than through the government, I think. The advantages of having a broad-based therapeutic that crosses several potential bioterrorist agents, as Dr. Thomas mentioned, for example, offers an advantage in that regard, in the sense that there's a larger market for it. If you had a very narrow-targeted therapeutic, the commercial market and big pharma would be less interested.

Dr. WELDON. So if it's got a clinical application, and it's in the treatment of cancer, for example——

Dr. FRIEDLANDER. Yes.

Dr. WELDON [continuing]. It could make it very easy to bring something like this to market? Based on the testimony we heard in the first panel, I think there's some real potential clinical applications in treating other diseases with the use of these products.

Would both of you say the level of funding, excusing you from this question, has been adequate so far for the type of research that needs to be done in this arena? I guess you don't really want to answer that either because you work for the Federal Government, right?

Mr. LEPPLA. Yes.

Mr. BALHORN. Well, I do, too.

Dr. WELDON. Oh, you work for the Federal Government also? OK, well, forget about that question then.

Well, I want to thank all of you. I will yield to the gentleman from Connecticut for questioning.

Mr. SHAYS. Thank you. Mr. Chairman, I'm usually not speechless, but at this hearing I have been, and I'm not sure if it was I needed more sleep or just was not catching on quickly to the dialog or compelling myself to. Maybe it was some of my old classes that came back to haunt me here, the memory of them. I felt like I was back in school.

I guess what I'm trying to think of is the bottom line for me is that we have the potential that anthrax could be used as a weapon against our military forces or our community at large, and that we need, in the case of not providing a prophylactic of vaccine, that we need to treat, and be able to effectively treat, those who have contracted anthrax.

Now, Dr. Friedlander, I'm well aware of the government's program to basically vaccine, and I do have my differences with that program. But what I'm interested to know from the three of you, and I would have asked the earlier panel, if I had gotten back in time, I want to know your reaction when you started to see that we were under attack by anthrax—letters, shutting down, we shut down a government building. My building was shut down for 5 weeks. We shut down another government building for 3 months. There was even talk at one point, and it was serious, that there was even question whether they would have to tear down the building. I mean, that's absurd, but it was real-live talk. Then we began to wonder the potential of what we were looking at.

So I want to know how you reacted and what clicked in, and did you say, you know, we've got some answers here? Are we seeing the ingenuity of the American people at work in what we've seen in the previous panel and this panel? So walk me through some of the things that I can grasp a little better.

Why don't we start with you, Mr. Balhorn? How did you react when you started to see this happen?

Mr. BALHORN. Well, I think probably my first reaction, and probably the same reaction that many people have, was those of us that have sort of thought about this and worked in this area for a number of years were never totally convinced that biological weapons could actually, or would actually, be used. There was always some concern about it's a threat that we worry about, but there wasn't any certainty associated with it.

I think a lot of us that understand the biochemistry, the biology of this, of these agents, also know how easy it is to do this. So the event itself showed that we really are in a new world, that biological weapons are a serious threat.

Mr. SHAYS. Let me just say, easy for you, but, I mean, some of what we heard was that this was sophisticated, not easy to do, and therefore—so put it in what context. It is easy——

Mr. BALHORN. Well, I guess easy in the context of designing—it's probably not a good example, but say if you wanted to develop a nuclear weapon, there are certain things you would have to have. Plutonium is one of them. It's difficult to get. It's something that's fairly limited and complicated and takes certain experts to deal with.

In biology you have the same field of—you know, you have expertise. But we've progressed in teaching even our students certain aspects in biology that they can carry out as college students or even high school students in some special courses. A lot of these things are what can be, what are used to produce some of these compounds, just growing bacteria in culture and isolating spores, things like that.

So in that concept——

Mr. SHAYS. Easy, OK.

Mr. BALHORN. In that respect.

So I think the main thing was that it convinced me and others that it is a real threat and there needs to be a concerted effort to minimize those specific types of threat agents that might be used.

Mr. SHAYS. But, I mean, when the Twin Towers were hit after having 19 hearings on terrorism, I found myself, as the buildings were going down or shortly afterwards, saying to myself out loud, my gosh, there's no red line; there's no line that terrorists won't cross.

Mr. BALHORN. That's right.

Mr. SHAYS. So they answered the one question that I had wondered: Would they use biological chemicals, potentially nuclear weapons? And the answer was a hearty yes; a very frightened yes is the way I should say it.

But now you're an expert in this field, and things didn't actually unfold the way we anticipated. For instance, under the program the military had, we were going to vaccinate everyone because my committee had been told continually that inhaled anthrax was death; there was no cure; there was no way to deal with it.

So what was happening here? I mean, we did cure people who had inhaled it. So what happened?

Mr. BALHORN. Well, I think Dr. Friedlander could probably answer that better than I could.

Mr. SHAYS. But what happened in your own mind? Were you surprised that all of a sudden we were able to deal with inhaled anthrax?

Mr. BALHORN. No, I wasn't. I mean, I'm aware that you can be infected by a variety of pathogens and there are treatments for them. It often depends on how you contract it, the level that the organism is reproduced to before you actually get treated, and the susceptibility of the individual. Every individual is slightly more susceptible.

Mr. SHAYS. I don't know where you were in our hearings, but one of the whole justifications for the military's program of vaccination was that we on this side of the table were being irresponsible to suggest that there not be a vaccination program, because if you contracted anthrax through a weaponized program of inhaling it, that you were dead. So you're telling me you're not surprised. I was surprised, but I'm not an expert, only because I listened to the experts who told me I should be surprised.

Mr. BALHORN. I guess probably there are very few things where you with certainty can say that, if you are exposed to it in terms of biological, that it will kill you for certain, because of the way individuals respond and the conditions under which they contract it.

Mr. SHAYS. Well, we lost five people. So five people did die from it.

Mr. BALHORN. Yes, right. So, yes, I was surprised at such a small number.

Mr. SHAYS. Yes.

Mr. BALHORN. But what went through my mind was that we can accelerate the pace; we need to, and that although there were fewer people—you know, more people survived than we thought. I think we were very lucky.

Mr. SHAYS. Yes, I kind of tuned out when you were taking the diagrams and when the first panel was here. I apologize, but I kind of did. But I was trying to think of the bottom line. The bottom line is, though, that both panels—and I would like to come to the next two panelists—the bottom line was that we were talking more of a cure rather than a prophylactic, is that correct?

Mr. BALHORN. Not necessarily, because many of these compounds can be used as a prophylactic, where you could, if you expect someone might have been exposed recently, they could be treated in advance.

Mr. SHAYS. OK, well, but they were exposed. In other words, so there's an interim. In other words, there's a prophylactic before it catches on?

Mr. BALHORN. Right.

Mr. SHAYS. OK. But, in other words, we're not going to vaccinate all the American people.

Mr. BALHORN. Right.

Mr. SHAYS. We're not even going to vaccinate all the military forces, I don't believe.

Mr. BALHORN. Right.

Mr. SHAYS. Unless we develop a new vaccine. But if we suspect—and the bottom line is we can pretty much determine if someone's been exposed? It was kind of curious, I'd just say this to you: You know, we were asking people to come and be tested on whether they had contracted anthrax, and the place we invited them to go was the Hart Building. I told my staff, I said, you know, be tested; don't go there; that's crazy.

Mr. BALHORN. Well, one of the difficulties is being able to detect with certainty that they've been exposed, because the symptoms, the very early symptoms, are a lot like flu. So I think one of the things that is difficult in this case is they can progress to a certain stage before the individual is aware.

But there are a variety of new technologies that are being developed where you can detect infections. The DNA-based technologies have been around for quite some time, allowing us to detect the organism. In some cases, or in many cases actually, when an individual takes a chemical into their body or they are infected by an organism, their body produces antibodies; they start producing them fairly quickly. Once people are starting to use those technologies of looking for the antibodies that are present, or the products that the cell produces in response to the presence of the organism—so, currently, I don't know of any method where we can detect shortly after someone's been exposed.

Mr. SHAYS. I want to go on to the next panelist, but there's so many hearings that we've had on this, and you just trigger one thing after another. I mean, for us and our panel, when we were looking at anthrax as a prophylactic to our military, we were basically told, this is the story; this is the way it is, and this is what we've got to do. Iraq has weaponized anthrax. Our troops are going to be in that theater. We have to protect them.

Yet, you were working before, and working after, September 11th dealing with anthrax, experimenting with it, correct? Or aren't I correct?

Mr. BALHORN. Me personally?

Mr. SHAYS. Yes.

Mr. BALHORN. No, we have not. So what we're doing is we're designing reagents for detecting botulinum toxin, but we've moving on to anthrax, yes.

Mr. SHAYS. OK. Mr. Leppla, or Doctor, I want to know how you responded to September 11th. I want to know if you were involved in the anthrax program before September 11th at all. I want to know what your reaction was when you saw these letters going out. I want to know what you suspected. I just want to know your reaction.

Mr. LEPPLA. Well, as an intramural researcher at NIH, I have been working on very basic aspects of anthrax toxin for 20 years, initially at USAMRIID and then at NIH. But NIH, of course, is not a front-line responder to public health emergencies.

Mr. SHAYS. Right.

Mr. LEPPLA. So there were no immediate changes in our activities. I was called occasionally for advice on reagent availability and things like this, but I haven't had a role in responding to the emergency aspects of this. NIH traditionally has looked for medical therapies, and in this case I think has not traditionally had a role in vaccine development for anthrax, but has now, of course, mounted that.

Mr. SHAYS. What did you think of the military's program to vaccinate every person in the military, whether or not they were going to be in a theater under threat?

Mr. LEPPLA. That's a policy issue that's well beyond my area of expertise. I mean, I have worked with the protective antigens for many years. So it's my understanding, and view from reading the publicly available literature, that the vaccine has been carefully evaluated by the FDA. So I thought the DOD was certainly on reasonable grounds in deciding to administer this licensed vaccine to the military.

Mr. SHAYS. No troubles on the fact that military personnel were required to do it, even under threat of being dishonorably discharged?

Mr. LEPPLA. Well, again, that's an area beyond my——

Mr. SHAYS. Do you work for, are you working for the government now?

Mr. LEPPLA. I work for the NIH.

Mr. SHAYS. Is that why you're reluctant to answer the question?

Mr. LEPPLA. It's——

Mr. SHAYS. I'm going to respect your reason, but I'm dumbfounded by it, why someone who obviously has expertise would not have an opinion.

Mr. LEPPLA. Well, my expertise is in basic research. I mean, I do have a—and I'm not involved in any way in evaluating the vaccine or I don't have access to the data that the DOD has collected on——

Mr. SHAYS. Well, we had people who were much more inquisitive than you sitting before us in previous hearings. We've had some people who have suggested that their biggest concern—we asked one individual who is an editor of a major medical magazine, a doctor, we asked him what was the question we should have asked him, and he said, well, my biggest concern is that a cottage industry operation of a few scientists could develop a biological agent that had been altered to the point that there would be no antidote and that we could wipe out mankind as we know it. That was a pretty strong statement for someone. He didn't need to say that, but he said it because he felt that we should know that's a real concern.

When you know that, you then say, well, I understand maybe why we make arrests, why we might have tribunals, why we're calling this a war, and why we're working as hard as we can to shut down the terrorists before they annihilate the human race. I'm just curious as to what your—I'm not a scientist; you are—whether you had similar emotions or whether you kind of yawned and said, well, you know, this doesn't seem to be all that big a deal. What was your reaction? When you saw letters that saw anthrax and buildings of the government being shut down, and a question mark on whether we had run out of anthrax as a vaccine, what was going through your mind?

Mr. LEPPLA. Well, of course, I had all the same concerns of any other citizen, but in terms of my job responsibilities, it was not something that was part of my job function. So as a witness here representing in some way NIH, I'm not sure that my personal views are——

Mr. SHAYS. OK, I'm going to respect that.

Dr. Friedlander——

Dr. FRIEDLANDER. Yes?

Mr. SHAYS [continuing]. Thank you for your service to your country. Our spontaneous applause is heartfelt, and that you would spend your last day with this committee is probably one of the highest compliments you could pay us. [Laughter.]

I would like to just ask you a few questions. I would like to ask you how confident you are about data from animal studies about the safety and efficacy of vaccines and anti-toxins in humans.

Dr. FRIEDLANDER. I think it's prudent to look at all the data that one has in trying to make an assessment. As someone alluded to earlier, for some diseases it's very difficult to test in the human population. So you have to take a look at all the best data that you have and come up with the best medical assessment as to the risk and the benefit.

Mr. SHAYS. When I was growing up and they were developing a small pox vaccine, polio, and so on, we would basically test it on animals and then humans, animals first to determine safety, and then humans to determine efficacy, and we could determine that there would be some population that a certain percentage would contract the disease. Therefore, we could then begin to know the efficacy of particular vaccines. But we don't have that, the ability to do this in this kind of instance, do we?

Dr. FRIEDLANDER. That's correct, and I think the FDA is trying to deal with that in the best way that they can. I don't know the current status of that, but——

Mr. SHAYS. But it does suggest to me, not being a scientist, obviously, but that any universal requirement to take a vaccine that hasn't been tested in terms of efficacy with humans, you really have to be very cautious, correct?

Dr. FRIEDLANDER. Well, I think that's correct, and I think the same argument holds with any therapeutic drug that's being considered for the same diseases.

Mr. SHAYS. What was your reaction when you saw what was happening with anthrax? You've heard the question I've asked. Walk me through September, after September 11th, and how you reacted.

Dr. FRIEDLANDER. Well, I think the world changed, and I think there was a sense of urgency, a sense of concern that was unprecedented, and involving the CDC and I think NIH, as well as DOD.

Mr. SHAYS. When we talk about the five people who have been literally murdered from anthrax being sent in the mail, this weaponized anthrax, tell me how we and how you work through the fact that we are part of the Biological Weapons Convention of 1972, and in there the protocol is very clear: Offensive use of biological agents is prohibited; any research for offensive use is prohibited, but defensive is not.

So you have been involved in, obviously, on the defensive side of biological agents. You do have to create the weapon, though, to know how to defend against it. Just walk me through the challenge that exists.

Dr. FRIEDLANDER. I'm not sure I can do that. I've not been involved in any research along those lines. It's been geared over the years——

Mr. SHAYS. Are you indirectly involved?

Dr. FRIEDLANDER. No.

Mr. SHAYS. So Fort Detrick does not get involved in anything of that——

Dr. FRIEDLANDER. I can't speak for Fort Detrick.

Mr. SHAYS. Are we walking on sensitive ground in terms of classified versus non-classified?

Dr. FRIEDLANDER. No, I think you have to address that with the Medical Research and Materiel Command.

Mr. SHAYS. So you haven't been involved in any way with the anthrax program?

Dr. FRIEDLANDER. No, that's not what I said, no. I have been, but only from the perspective of developing countermeasures.

Mr. SHAYS. Well, then, walk me through that. Walk me through that.

Dr. FRIEDLANDER. Specifically——

Mr. SHAYS. Yes. Tell me what kinds of things you've been required to do.

Dr. FRIEDLANDER. Well, I started working on anthrax a long time ago, when we were——

Mr. SHAYS. One of the reasons why I'm asking the question, obviously, is that there's concern that the anthrax that we've had to deal with has been anthrax that may have been developed by our own personnel, be they military or not, and obviously an aberration, someone who's simply taken their solemn responsibilities and flipped it on end and turned against our own country. But walk me through it.

Mr. Chairman, do I have 5 more minutes?

Mr. BURTON [resuming Chair]. I beg your pardon?

Mr. SHAYS. Do I have 5 more minutes?

Mr. BURTON. Sure, we'll give you 5 more minutes. I have another meeting I want to go to, and I'm going to ask one question.

Mr. SHAYS. Well, I'm going to just then yield to you.

Mr. BURTON. OK, and then what I'll do is I'll let you have the Chair and then you can finish in 5 minutes.

Mr. SHAYS. Yes, and I'll be finished, so I won't keep them much longer.

Mr. BURTON. I just have one question, and that is for you, Dr. Friedlander. I'm sorry to lose you. I hear you're retiring, and I hear you have done very fine things for this country. So I wish you the best for the future.

Dr. FRIEDLANDER. Thank you.

Mr. BURTON. We've heard that anthrax spores used in the mail attacks that we dealt with here on Capitol Hill originated at Fort Detrick. Do you have any information whatsoever about that?

Dr. FRIEDLANDER. No. I think that's an issue for the FBI so far as I know.

Mr. BURTON. For the FBI?

Dr. FRIEDLANDER. It's my understanding that they're investigating, they're in charge of the investigation——

Mr. BURTON. Is the military doing anything like investigating whether or not there were any leaks or anybody down there that was previous personnel that might have been involved in that?

Dr. FRIEDLANDER. I'm not involved in that at all. So far as I know, the FBI is in charge of the investigation.

Mr. BURTON. OK, very good.

Mr. Shays, can you take the chair then?

Oh, let me just, before I leave, because I'm going to turn the Chair over to Mr. Shays and he can conclude the meeting, I hope that you will remember what I suggested to the first panel. That is, any ideas that you have on what should be done in the area of funding, research, creating research teams, or anything that needs to be done to speed up the process of coming up with countermeasures or vaccines or other substances to ward off chemical or biological attacks, we'd like to have that submitted to our committee, in addition to NIH.

I know NIH is looking at this, and I know they're working very diligently to come up with these vaccines and countermeasures, but one of the reasons I'm asking for that, and I think Mr. Shays would like to have it, as well as the rest of the committee, is we're the ones that help get the funding for these various research projects. Because time is of the essence, we need to have that information, so that we can make a determination on how much money is necessary, and if we have to go to the President and ask him to go along with additional appropriations for this research, we want to do that, because we don't want to be caught flat-footed if there's an attack. OK? So if you could get that for us, we would really appreciate it.

Mr. Shays.

Mr. SHAYS [assuming Chair]. Can I just sit here with the gavel?

Mr. BURTON. If you'd like, I'll throw it to you.

Mr. SHAYS. No, don't throw it. [Laughter.]

Because I'm not going to be that long. Thank you, Mr. Chairman. Thank you, sir.

Dr. Friedlander, this is a serious question. It is trying to understand how one divides, knows when they are doing defensive versus offensive. In order to do defensive—and let me just preface something, so you don't try to anticipate something you don't need to anticipate.

I happen to believe in the protocol of 1972. I also happen to believe in the administration's rejection of the Convention that somehow attempted to allow for surveillance in a way that I thought was ineffective that was rejected this last fall with a variety of nations. It was too ironic for me that Iran and Iraq were part of the Convention that was trying to determine how we were going to oversee the potential of offensive use of chemical weapons, and the hypocrisy of that was more than I could stand.

But tell me what you do. You take anthrax that is produced by our country. It has to be weaponized and then you try to determine how you deal with this weaponized anthrax? All I'm trying to understand is, you have to make the weapon in order to know how to defend against it, isn't that true?

Dr. FRIEDLANDER. I think that's true.

Mr. SHAYS. Yes.

Dr. FRIEDLANDER. I mean, I'm not sure, I think the research that's been ongoing has—there has not been—I'm not sure that work, in terms of the evaluation of vaccines, for example, that we've done over the years at USAMRIID has used anthrax spores to test essentially.

Mr. SHAYS. But has some of what has been discussed today been actively pursued in your facilities?

Dr. FRIEDLANDER. Some of the approaches to treatment you mean?

Mr. SHAYS. Yes, yes.

Dr. FRIEDLANDER. Some of them have, yes.

Mr. SHAYS. But, in order to do that, you have to deal with an aerosoled anthrax, correct?

Dr. FRIEDLANDER. Yes.

Mr. SHAYS. Yes. So can I make an assumption that, if we think a particular country is developing a particular type of weaponized biological agent, that we have to take that weaponized biological agent in order to know how to respond defensively to it?

Dr. FRIEDLANDER. Well, I can't quite answer that. I mean, there may be some differences. The ways in which we test it are by aerosolizing liquid spores, and that's different than what was in the envelopes.

Mr. SHAYS. You mean that particular——

Dr. FRIEDLANDER. The method of producing spores.

Mr. SHAYS. OK, refresh me. How was the method——

Dr. FRIEDLANDER. Well, we use the liquid formulation in the testing of vaccines and antibiotics, for example.

Mr. SHAYS. Let me just ask each of the panelists—first, preface it by saying, I have a basic theory that if you unleash American or just human ingenuity, but it seems best in the United States because we seem to unleash it better, that when we're confronted with challenges, that we, through the private, public, government sectors, can sometimes find very clever, very simple responses to what we thought were impossible tasks before people began to think it through.

The reason, my motivation in asking you what you were thinking was, did you all come and say, after September 11th, and after you started seeing what we were faced with as a country, did you start to redesign your activities and your research and your thought process to say, you know, we can make a contribution here? That's the assumption I have made. Is that an incorrect assumption?

Mr. BALHORN. My answer is yes, because I'll give you one example. The technologies that we were developing, are developing, or are using, they haven't changed as a result of that event, but what has changed is the fact that what we were developing and are currently funded for are detection reagents, the first line of defense, trying to find out where it is, who's been exposed to it, and so forth.

But what convinced me, what I was convinced of after that was that we really could apply the same methods to development of therapeutics to save those people that were exposed. So it did have an impact, and I think it's something that—well, basically, that's it.

Mr. SHAYS. So then one of the reasons why we are having this hearing was to put on the record a response and give it some attention. That's been part of the motivation of this hearing. One of the things that is troubling to me as a Member of Congress is that there's probably two or three people a week, sometimes one, sometimes more than three—and when I say "people," organizations, groups of people—who come to me and say they have an answer for this particular problem, whether it's detecting explosives on planes. We are becoming a little frustrated—I don't like to use that word often—because we refer them to whom? We refer them to the Office on Homeland Security, and we know that's becoming a bottomless pit, of which there's no capacity yet to know and evaluate good ideas and bad ideas, to know what are bad and reject and what are good and accept.

One of the things that concerns me is, and one of the reasons we're having this hearing, I think, is to make sure that we are a force that is contributing to catching these good ideas and seeing how they can be implemented.

Dr. Leppla, are you being asked to evaluate a lot of different private sector ideas? Are you having more people contact you? What's happened that's different in your life since September 11th?

Mr. LEPPLA. Certainly a great deal is different, yes. I mean, I often say anthrax was an orphan disease in the middle eighties when a few of us were working on it, not very many people were aware of it, or considered it a significant problem. Clearly, the situation is very different now.

I'm one person in the field, but I'm still getting many calls from academics or small companies or large companies who wish to contribute in some way to research on anthrax therapies. Many of these have very impressive technologies. The NIAID hasn't, although I'm not a member of the NIAID, they clearly have been very responsive in putting out a number of new funding opportunities. I know just in the last month two deadlines have passed for submission of both SBIR and RO–1 grants from universities. My impression is they've had tremendous response to those requests for proposals.

So a great many people out there are wanting to contribute, and I'm glad in a little way to be able to advise them or provide them with reagents. So things are very different.

Mr. SHAYS. Thank you.

With the power invested in me here, I'm going to invite anyone who was in the previous panel, if they have a closing comment that they want to make, any last thought that they would like to make, and I would also invite—is there anyone from the previous panel that wishes we had asked a question that they had prepared to answer and not been able to answer it because they weren't asked?

And anyone on this panel that would like to ask a question that we didn't ask that they would like to answer?

First, let me start with that: Is there anyone on this panel that has a question that they would like to ask themselves and then answer, that you'd like to put on the record? I'm not trying to be cute, but that you'd like to put on the record. Is there anything else?

Mr. BALHORN. Well, I'd like to make a comment and sort of echo—a couple of comments of what Dr. Friedlander said. You've asked a number of questions about the vaccine and the difficulties associated with that. I think it's important to point out and reiterate that any drug or treatment that we develop has to go through the same kind of testing, and can have potential problems. So by talking about designing, even using computers, molecules that bind the special sites, and they only bind to one protein, in practice that turns out not to be the case and they have to be tested.

So these things also, I think it's important to say, take time, not that it has to take 10 to 12 years to accomplish what you want. It can take a few years, but it's not something that can be done in 6 months or 8 months. So I think it's really important that you and your committee have an impact on basically the basic science and funding for the basic science that needs to go into this.

Anthrax is the first one that you're considering, but there are a number of potential targets or agents that can be used as bioweapons. A lot of the methods we've talked about translate directly into producing, you know, inhibitors for those as well.

So I think it's really important to think ahead. We've seen that bioweapons will be used. They may not come back and use the same one next time. So we need to think a little bit about what are the next potential ones and put an effort toward solving those.

What you worry about is that there are a lot of different agents. You can also keep in mind, help yourself in terms of working toward that is that all of these agents are actually threats to the community outside bioterrorism. In some cases like anthrax it's a very small threat, but you've talked about Ebola. That's a threat that shows up repeatedly as well. So I think there's a benefit of that, besides the applications to things like cancer research.

Mr. SHAYS. Some of the most impressive meetings that I've had overseas have been with the World Health Organization and people who literally go to very dangerous spots in the world, not knowing what kind of pathogen they're dealing with, but they go there, in some cases I feel unarmed and unprotected, to try to understand what's happening.

One of the things in my previous work as chairman of the Human Resources Committee overseeing HHS and CDC, and so on, is the incredible new threats that may develop that aren't manmade but just a result of human contact and interaction, and so on. What I wrestle with, as a public official, is the ethics of the government mandating vaccines where we know that there will always be some that will respond in a negative way, and then what obligation do we have to those who respond negatively? In other words, there's always going to be a certain percentage, and the fact that they are under command and under threat of court marshall, and the concept that seems to be evolving in some of the military, that we are going to protect our military by just injecting them with more vaccines. So we all are wrestling with a lot of things.

But the one thing I am pretty certain of is there's a lot of ingenuity out in our country, and there's a lot we can learn. I'm just hoping that the government has the ability to accept good ideas and reject bad ones. It used to be the large ate the small; now it's the fast eat the slow. I don't think our government can move quickly sometimes.

So, Dr. Friedlander, do you have any other comment that you would like to make?

Dr. FRIEDLANDER. No, thank you.

Mr. SHAYS. I do appreciate your being here very much.

Dr. FRIEDLANDER. Thank you.

Mr. SHAYS. Is there anyone from the other panel that would like to make a closing comment?

[No response.]

If not, we'll call this hearing adjourned. Thank you very much.

[Whereupon, at 1:35 p.m., the committee was adjourned, to reconvene at the call of the Chair.]

[The prepared statement of Hon. Wm. Lacy Clay follows:]

Statement of the Honorable William Lacy Clay
Before the
Government Reform Committee
February 28, 2002

"Quickening the Pace of Research in Protecting against Anthrax and Other Biological Terrorist Agents – A Look at Toxin Interference"

Mr. Chairman, I would like to preface my remarks by stating that I am in full support of continued medical research that will protect the lives of Americans against anthrax and other biological threats. If quickening the pace of medical research helps save lives then I am committed to asking for additional funding from Congress to make that happen.

However, I would urge that we err on the side of caution before new products are released to the American public for consumption. Appropriate testing by the FDA and USDA must first take place in order to ensure public safety.

I would like to recommend the establishment of a new partnership between various government agencies such as the National Institutes of Health (NIH), - America's leading research labs, colleges and universities to develop new techniques to fight bio-terrorism.

By accelerating the research in order to provide added protection, more harm than good could occur. The very medicines that are supposed to help save lives may in fact, become the ones that hurt a greater number of people without proper testing controls.

One thing is for certain-time is of the essence. Bio-terrorist who would do harm to the American public are not waiting for this panel to make decisions about speeding up the research process. This Committee must act in an expedient manner and commit all of its resources in our fight against the bio-terrorism threat. I am pleased that this hearing was called to address this important issue. We must now look to the future for answers.

Mr. Chairman, I ask unanimous consent to submit my remarks to the record.

APEX
TP
9780160685507
76901945 — 45